Fit for Fligh

MW01678527

Fit for Flight

Flight Physiology and Human Factors for Aircrew

SECOND EDITION

Richard O. Reinhart, MD

Iowa State University Press / Ames

RICHARD O. REINHART, MD, is a senior FAA Aviation Medical Examiner and retired Air National Guard Flight Surgeon. An instrument-rated commercial pilot and president of Human Factors Resources, Inc., Reinhart is a contributing editor to *Business & Commercial Aviation* and author of several books, including *FAA Medical Certification.*

© 1999 Iowa State University Press
All rights reserved

First edition © 1993 TAB Books, *Fit to Fly: A Pilot's Guide to Health & Safety*

Iowa State University Press
2121 South State Avenue, Ames, Iowa 50014

Orders:	1-800-862-6657
Office:	1-515-292-0140
Fax:	1-515-292-3348
Web site:	www.isupress.edu

Although care has been taken to ensure the accuracy of this book, it is not a substitute for medical advice. Always consult your own doctor; the author and publisher cannot take responsibility for your health.

Authorization to photocopy items for internal or personal use, or the internal or personal use of specific clients, is granted by Iowa State University Press, provided that the base fee of $.10 per copy is paid directly to the Copyright Clearance Center, 222 Rosewood Drive, Danvers, MA 01923. For those organizations that have been granted a photocopy license by CCC, a separate system of payments has been arranged. The fee code for users of the Transactional Reporting Service is 0-8138-1567-3/99 $.10.

♾ Printed on acid-free paper in the United States of America

First edition, 1993
Second edition, 1999

International Standard Book Number: 0-8138-1567-3

Library of Congress Cataloging-in-Publication Data

Reinhart, Richard O.
Fit for flight : flight physiology and human factors for aircrew / Richard O. Reinhart.—2nd ed.
p. cm.
Prev. ed. published with title: Fit to fly.
Includes bibliographical references and index.
ISBN 0-8138-1567-3
1. Flight—Physiological aspects. 2. Aviation medicine.
I. Reinhart, Richard O. Fit to fly. II. Title.
RC1075.R455 1999
616.9′80213—dc21 99–27343

The last digit is the print number: 9 8 7 6 5 4 3 2 1

Contents

Introduction

Oh, I have slipped the surly bonds of earth
And danced the skies on laughter silvered wings;
Sunward I've climbed and joined the tumbling mirth
Of sun split clouds and done a hundred things
You have not dreamed of ...

IT SOUNDS MAGICAL, but ask any pilot how to fly an airplane in three words and the response will probably be: needle, ball, and airspeed. These are the fundamentals of flying. As your hours build, each flight becomes a new training experience. Hours of dual and solo practice make you proficient, and learning commercial maneuvers, instrument flight, and the ultimate ATP rating round you out as the complete pilot—ready for anything that's thrown your way. Yet, the more you dance around the skies, the more you realize that although flying may rely on a few basics, you are not invulnerable to other variables. Just as the aircraft is subject to mechanical factors, you the pilot are subject to "human factors." You are probably not even aware of all of these human factors nor of the profound effect they can have on your flying skills.

You have discovered that simply knowing how to move the stick and rudder does not make you a safe or proficient pilot. As you gain experience, you realize that the more you know about the stick and rudder, airfoils, engines, hydraulics, and also weather, the better and safer pilot you will be. The same holds true with understanding *how* your body and mind can be affected in flight as well as *why* you are affected. I can preach human factors, health, and flight physiology, but until you actually feel and sense these effects, you will have little respect for the outcome. Furthermore, it is common for many physiological situations to be occurring at the same time, not a very comforting thought if you aren't even aware of what's happening!

In earlier days, pilots on TV and in the movies were often

fearless, overcoming great odds in dangerous skies. They were flying planes that were falling apart as they neared their fateful destination. They knew, however, that they could rise above the inadequacies of their mind, body, and machine. Even today, macho pilots believe they can drink up a storm, stagger out of the bar, and fly a perfect trip the next day. They pass off the effects of fatigue, dehydration, noise, hypoglycemia, and the myriad of other factors associated with flight. Could you be in this group—even occasionally? If so, then it is definitely time for you to improve your understanding of human factors because they are often the symptoms behind the finding of pilot error.

As aviation becomes a major part of our lives, the subject of human factors goes beyond those in the cockpit. The same stresses affect individuals in the cabin: the flight attendants and passengers. Although this book focuses on the primary crew (pilots), the cabin crew also needs to understand much of what is discussed herein. The term *flightcrew* addresses this team effort, especially as noted in any crew resource management (CRM) training. This concept was once called *"cockpit" resource management* until it was recognized that the flight attendants played a key role in flight safety and that their performance also was affected by human factors and flight physiology. Therefore, even though "pilot" is frequently used, "flight attendant" can be often substituted in the discussions.

The objective for you as the reader is to get a clear understanding and overview of the many and varied physiological situations that can interfere with your safe flight. The military has long been the expert in flight physiology. This manual is not meant to reinvent the wheel but it does reiterate some material already presented in military publications. You are constructed the same way as military pilots so the information is generic for everyone that takes to the skies. This manual is also meant to be a resource in your personal flying library. Situations dealing with human factors and flight physiology will occur and it's easier for you to refer to your own resources rather than depend on someone else's war story or uninformed answer.

When it comes to hypoxia, disorientation, jet lag, vision problems, etc., some pilots and flight attendants don't even know what these terms mean, and many don't care. Many aircrew members have little access to resources providing this insight. This situation doesn't mean that these issues are less important than flight proficiency or learning how to fly an ILS. They may not be as exciting or as challenging as sharpening your flying skills. But, they will all have a direct or indirect affect on your flight and performance skills—and you may not even be aware of what and why your skills are compromised. You may be the best pilot on the field, but not if you allow yourself to be subjected to and affected by the physiological factors that literally surround all flightcrew.

Flight physiology and human factors both have an impact on flight. Over 70 percent of aviation accidents and incidents is in some way related to human factors. Do you know when to say, "I'm not safe!"? Do you fully understand hypoxia, fatigue, or the effects of self-medication? That's the purpose of this book. To help you understand the other part of flight—the human part—and to recognize when your body or mind is not in tune with the aircraft.

We all would like to fly in ideal conditions, with good weather, working radios, no delays, functioning instruments, and propellers turning. No flight is ideal, however. Furthermore, your mind and body may not fully cooperate during a problem flight when all your physical and mental skills are needed. Now you become prime for an incident or accident. Flying an approach to minimums with a faltering engine and an intermittent glide slope is stressful, but you probably can deal with the situation. If you are fatigued, disoriented, or suffering with an ear block, however, your approach to minimums may be downright dangerous!

The Human Factors of Safe Flight

Human factors has a variety of definitions, depending on who you ask. A psychologist defines it as how you deal with stress, how you communicate with crewmates and ATC, how you manage the variety of resources available to you in a critical situation (i.e., CRM). A physiologist or physician expects you to be familiar with the effects of fatigue, hypoglycemia, illness, noise, and other medical issues. You may say it means the ability to perform under extreme conditions, or how you judge what action to take when things turn sour. The objective is the same. How to get you, your passengers, and your airplane from point A to point B in a normally functioning flying machine without the interference of a human factor.

Flight physiology is how your body and mind work in the flying environment. It includes understanding how your organs function, what keeps them from functioning, and what you can do to protect these functions before and during flight. Hypoxia, dehydration, fatigue, vibration, visual illusions, noise, disorientation, jet lag, self-medication, alcohol, smoking, and many more are included under flight physiology. And this list is growing as the aviation community recognizes more factors. Furthermore, how to define your health and how to protect your health become important goals. Flight physiology may not be as exciting as learning how to make perfect landings, but it is not dull, nor is it just something that is nice to know. Nor should crisis management be the initiative to learn. It is essential to safe flight. Ask any pilot who has been disoriented or incapacitated with an ear block.

We take these issues for granted because our bodies and minds are usually tolerant and forgiving of the abuses to which we subject them. Just once in a while, don't you think that human factors happen only to the other pilot and that he or she should have known better? Denial of the importance of human factors compared with flight proficiency begins to take over our reasoning. The near hit or dumb incident usually gets our attention and brings us back to the reality of the significance of human factors. These are the pilots who don't have to be told to learn because they know its importance. The very fact that you are reading this manual suggests that you are, at the very least, curious about the human factors in flight.

Flight physiology, therefore, is an integral part of human factors and safe flight. We expect our aircraft to be airworthy. We look to our mechanics to keep our aircraft airworthy. Before you fly you preflight the machine to ensure that it is airworthy. Your expectations are high for your aircraft. You should have the same expectations for yourself and your flightcrew. They must also be airworthy—medically airworthy.

Safety is the prime goal of all flight for all pilots and flight attendants. Continue to read on. There may be some surprises and, at the least, a reinforcement of insight you learned years ago.

Are You Incapacitated?

When the first officer got the approach lights in sight, he informed the captain, adding that the aircraft was a little left of centerline. The deviation was so slight that he was not surprised when the captain did not immediately take corrective action. Some seconds later, with the runway less than 1 mile distant and the aircraft still left of centerline, he again made a remark to that effect. No immediate corrective action followed, but after a few seconds the aircraft turned slightly to the right and the crew assumed this was the expected correction. When, however, the turn continued and the aircraft crossed the centerline, both the second officer and the flight engineer simultaneously called for the first officer to take over. The first officer saw the captain's body lean forward in the shoulder harness, his right hand slipping slowly from the power levers. The height of the aircraft was approximately 150 feet. The first officer immediately took over full control and carried out a missed approach.

The ultimate objective of flight physiology awareness is the prevention of incapacitation, whether physical or mental. *Incapacitation* is defined as being incapable of, unfit or unable to perform normal activity. Mental incapacitation is your mind's inability to use proper judgment, reasoning, or thought processes. Mental incapacitation turns into neurological incapacitation when the signals from your brain fail to use the signals from your eyes and ears, and other sensory inputs from touch, smell, etc. Physical incapacitation refers to your body's inability to function in an expected way. The end result in any of these situations is an unsafe and poorly performing pilot.

Several types of incapacitation are recognized, all of which lead to the same unacceptable result—an unsafe pilot.

Sudden Incapacitation

The meaning of sudden incapacitation should be obvious. You may collapse or slump over the yoke. You may cry out in pain

A survey, originally conducted in 1967, and then repeated in 1988, revealed the following list of incapacitating symptoms as reported by professional pilots:

- Uncontrolled bowel action
- Nausea
- Vomiting
- Severe indigestion
- Earache
- Faintness
- Headache
- Nosebleed
- Toothache
- Eye injury
- Coughing attack
- Sneezing attack
- Leg or foot cramps

These still remain the causes of incapacitation.

or have a seizure. A solo pilot is committed to whatever the plane now chooses to do. With a crew, the others can take immediate action to keep the plane airborne—the first rule of safe flight in an emergency (fly the airplane!). Because the situation is usually so obvious, there is no doubt that something has to do be done and quickly. As a copilot, get the troubled pilot away from the controls and take over the flying, then declare an emergency and land. Do you feel you could determine if your crewmate is incapacitated and not in control and could you take over the controls without getting overly involved with the incapacitated pilot?

Subtle Incapacitation

Subtle incapacitation is less obvious. In fact, it can go unnoticed by you or your crewmates, which makes this type of incapacitation a potentially dangerous situation. It's like driving your car and not knowing your brakes are out—until you need them. You may be dazed, semiconscious, or unable to move (as with a stroke). What do you do if this is a senior pilot, your captain, or a check pilot? At what point do you take over without being charged with mutiny?

Total or Partial Incapacitation

Total incapacitation should be self-explanatory. There is no doubt that there is a problem that needs immediate attention. Partial incapacitation is more troublesome. Like with subtle incapacitation, you may not be aware of a deficiency. Or you

A good starting point. Most pilots give their aircraft a thorough preflight, yet many forget to preflight themselves. The "I'm Safe" checklist represents some of the topics to be covered in this manual and should be part of every pilot's flight preparation.

I*llness.*
Do I have any symptoms?

M*edication.*
Have I been taking prescription or OTC drugs?

S*afe.*
Am I under psychological pressure from my job? Do I have money, health, or family problems?

A*lcohol.*
Have I had anything to drink in the last 24 hours? Do I have a hangover?

F*atigue.* How much time has lapsed since my last flight?
Did I sleep well last night and am I adequately rested?

E*ating.*
Have I eaten enough of the proper foods to keep me adequately nourished during the entire flight?

The accident flight originated at 2:00 a.m. and terminated about 6:30 a.m. The 36-year-old pilot had an ATP rating and 7,500 hours. The accident investigation revealed the following problems and probable causes: Seven DUIs, driver's license revoked, drinking problems, three aircraft accidents, 20 traffic violations, incarcerations for DUI, two divorces, poor judgment, extreme fatigue, and hypoxia (i.e., human factors overload).

don't relate the reason you aren't performing well to being fatigued or sick with the flu, or something else. Regardless, you may not accept the realization that you are incapacitated and your pride forbids you from admitting this to yourself, your crewmates, or ATC. And if you aren't in the loop or admitting something is wrong, who is going to intervene?

Distraction

There is a place for the healthy pilot to be "kind of incapacitated" solely as a result of being distracted. This distraction can be caused by worrying about a problem at home, concentrating on a yellow warning light, listening to an unrelated conversation on the flight deck, and many other scenarios that take you out of the flying loop. Some call this a lack of situation awareness, not knowing or recognizing what's going on around you and your aircraft. Whatever the reason, distraction is always present and only you can get back on track—unless someone else brings your inattentiveness to your attention, like ATC. And, you are more susceptible to being distracted if you are physiologically affected.

Pride often gets in the way of resolving a situation before it turns into a crisis. Are you willing to admit you are having a problem, especially if you think you can deal with it yourself? If there is a slim chance that you are thinking that pride could get in your way, then this is another breakdown in use of cockpit and crew resources. Another unsafe situation occurs if you are unwilling to challenge another crewmate who is experiencing substandard performance, especially if you think it is possibly a result of some physiological problem. Assertiveness and self-confidence become important personality traits in good pilots and are key topics taught in CRM courses.

You aren't expected to be an expert in human factors and flight physiology. But I'm sure you agree that you must be aware of what can incapacitate you and your other crewmates who are occupying the same airspace. Crisis management results from being unprepared or unknowing. Take control of the controllable factors, the human factors discussed in this manual. Plan for incident prevention, not just accident prevention.

Fit for Flight SECOND EDITION

Your Challenges in Flight 1

"OFF WE GO, into the wild blue yonder, flying high into the sky." These words, from a popular Army Air Corps song written decades ago, express our desire to soar through the air with the birds. How often we wished we had wings. And, as everyone has heard, if God had meant us to fly, he would have given us wings. Really BIG wings! Because if you aren't flying with wings, how do you go off into the blue yonder?

We have to realize that there are three major parts to flight: the plane (or "aerospace vehicle"), the pilot (you), and the atmosphere (the environment in which you live and fly). There is an interrelationship between all three but it is the atmosphere that affects both the plane and the pilot, often in unpredictable ways. Whereas your airplane may be right at home in thin air, you are not. Your airplane's engine may be more efficient at altitude, but your body is not. This chapter helps explain the atmosphere and how your body functions within it.

Atmospheric Ingredients

The atmosphere is a gaseous envelope of air that surrounds the earth. It extends to about 25,000 miles above the surface of the earth. It rotates with the earth and its temperature and pressure are continuously changing. From a biological and physiological point of view, however, the composition of the atmosphere is constant. That is, no matter where you fly, the air is composed of the same relative kinds of gases. It's how much of these gases that is present, or their partial pressures, that concerns you.

There are a variety of layers of gases within the atmosphere (i.e., the troposphere, stratosphere, etc.), much like layers seen between water and oil (Fig. 1-1). The composition of air within each of these layers is different. These layers can be divided physiologically to identify where the dangers lie for pilots as

Fig. 1-1 The atmosphere is divided into layers based on temperature.

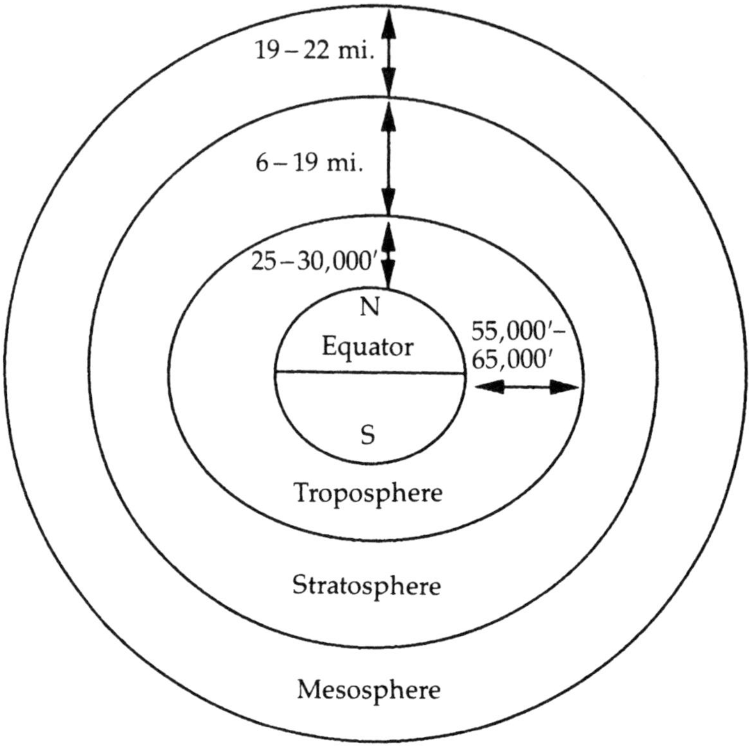

The composition of air within each of these layers is different. These layers can be divided physiologically to identify where the dangers lie for us as we fly from one elevation to another. All of these factors are directly related to known gas laws, which we all learned in high school. Understanding how your body is affected in these different layers is crucial to safe flight.

they fly from one elevation to another. All of these factors are directly related to known gas laws, something we all learned in high school. How your body is affected in these different layers is crucial to safe flight.

Because of changing gaseous amounts in the flight path, the composition of the atmosphere is expressed in percentages and not in absolute amounts. The percentage of oxygen (O_2) in the atmosphere is about 20 percent of the gases covering the earth. Yet the number of O_2 molecules, the actual amount of O_2 available to your body and all its parts, decreases with altitude. Furthermore, the percentages of these gases are slightly affected by the presence or absence of water vapor.

Of primary importance to you is the O_2 and nitrogen (N_2) you breathe and, to a lesser degree, carbon dioxide (CO_2), ozone (O_3), and water vapor. Too much or too little of any of these gases could not only compromise your health but also your safety. Your body is not very tolerant to variations in gas concentrations. Let's talk about each gas separately.

Oxygen

A colorless, odorless, tasteless elemental gas, O_2 is the most abundant of all elements on earth both in combination or by itself. It occurs as a free element in the atmosphere. Oxygen is roughly 20 percent of the total gases found in the atmosphere. The source of O_2 in our atmosphere is largely from the process of photosynthesis in which it is generated from carbon dioxide and water. Of all the gases, O_2 is the most essential in maintaining life. Any change in the O_2 levels that you breathe adversely affects how you fly. This effect is called hypoxia.

Nitrogen

Another colorless, odorless, tasteless elemental gas in the atmosphere is N_2. At 80 percent, it is the most plentiful gas in the atmosphere. Consequently, the major portion of the total atmospheric pressure or weight at and near the earth's surface is due to N_2. This gas can saturate the cells and tissues of your body and cause problems, such as the bends.

Carbon Dioxide

Although CO_2 makes up only 0.03 percent of the atmosphere, it creates some of the most disabling physiological problems, especially in flight. Like O_2 and N_2, CO_2 is also colorless, odorless, and tasteless. It is somewhat heavier than air and a byproduct of respiration. Because of our heavy use of fossil fuels for combustion, CO_2 is the only gaseous constituent of the atmosphere that has increased significantly during the past century.

Water Vapor

Water vapor is not considered one of the components of the atmosphere. When we talk about humidity and dew point we are talking about the water vapor in the air. The amount of water in the air around you depends on how much water remains as a gas (not as a liquid as in fog or clouds) as the temperature changes. Even at 100 percent humidity at 100°F, there is less than 5 percent water vapor relative to the other atmospheric gases. The percentage of water vapor decreases dramatically as you climb above the earth's surface. When you reach the stratosphere (see Fig. 1-1), the air is virtually dry.

Ozone

Ozone is an unstable, pale blue gas with a characteristic pungent odor often noticed around electrical equipment and in thunderstorms. It is found in high concentrations at altitudes greater than 5 miles above ground level. The ambient or surrounding O_3 concentration is dependent on the season, latitude, and altitude. Its concentration in the atmosphere is cyclic, changing its amount over many decades. Ozone is not considered a component of the atmosphere, it's found in the ionosphere.

The Physics of Gases

There are physical properties that are universally applied with any gas, especially a mixture of gases. The atmosphere is basically one large sack of gases surrounding the earth. These gases have a direct impact on how your body functions in flight.

Barometric or atmospheric pressure is the weight of all the molecules of the gases (the air) above you. Therefore, this weight, or pressure, decreases with altitude because there are fewer molecules (but in the same percentages). The pressure drop, however, is not linear because air is compressible. The density of a volume of air now plays a role in pressure change. The air near the surface of the earth is more dense, having more molecules of gases within a given volume, than air farther from the surface. Therefore, as you near the earth's surface, a greater pressure change occurs.

In addition to weight, there are a variety of physical properties of the atmosphere that affect barometric pressure, including temperature changes secondary to the seasons, weather systems, and your location on earth (the latitude and longitude). To establish a base pressure from which you can calculate your various pressures used in flight, a standard atmosphere must be defined. The most commonly used base is the international standard atmosphere (ISA), which establishes a mean atmospheric pressure of 29.92 inches of mercury, or 760 millimeters of mercury (mm Hg) at a temperature of 15°C (59°F) in dry air at sea level. If this sounds like needless information, it isn't if you recognize that all your flying colleagues need to be at the same pressure altitude—if they have corrected for these conditions and have their altimeters set correctly!

The earth's surface, as you know, is heated by the sun, which in turn re-radiates the heat into the air above ground. This radiation causes little heating of the atmosphere at higher elevations. As you ascend from the surface, the temperature falls steadily and predictably throughout the troposphere. This temperature lapse rate levels off at the tropopause (about 35,000 feet). Additionally, the tropopause is higher in the summer than in the winter, which means you will notice different outside air temperatures as you climb during each season.

Ninety-nine percent of the earth's atmosphere, in terms of the quantity of gases, exists below 20 miles (32 km). The greatest pressure change encountered is from sea level to about 5,000 feet. Therefore, even in a pressurized aircraft, such as an airliner, the problems associated with changes of pressure must be considered. Keep in mind that pressurized cabin altitudes often get up to 8,000 feet or more. That means you are hypoxic!

Physiologically, most pressures are expressed as standard atmospheric above sea level. Because you fly at varying altitudes, however, it is important to recognize that pressure is not constant. It is a variant of many physical properties, as explained in the gas laws you learned in school. The effects of pressure changes will become evident to you when I discuss the physiology of oxygen and carbon dioxide exchange in your body, pressure breathing at altitude, decompression sickness, and ear blocks.

Remember, the atmosphere is a mixture of gases and is subject to the gas laws of physics. If you are to understand how and why these gases affect your body, you also must have a basic understanding of these gas laws.

Boyle's Law states that the volume of a gas is inversely proportional to the pressure, with temperature remaining constant (Fig. 1-2). This law applies to all gases. In dealing with gas expansion in your body, however, a correction must be made for the ever-present water vapor. Such characteristics applied to your body explain the expansion of gases trapped in moist areas such as your middle ear, sinuses, stomach, and intestines. These are all actual or potential cavities within which moist air is present and/or can become trapped. Trapped gases are discussed later.

Because the atmosphere is a mixture of gases, and each gas has its own partial pressure at any given temperature within a

Fig. 1-2 Comparative volumes of dry gases at increasing altitude and decreasing pressure.

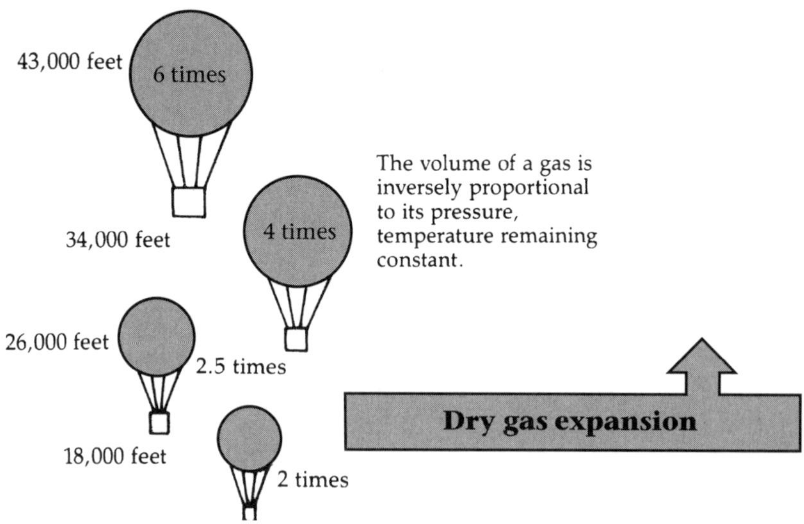

given volume, it is also important to know the physics of the combined pressures. *Dalton's Law* states that the total pressure of a gas mixture is the sum of the individual partial pressures that each gas would exert if it alone occupied the whole volume. Each kind of gas exerts its own partial pressure, depending on the percentage of that gas in the mixture. Thus, even though the percentage of O_2 in the atmosphere is constant (about 20%), its partial pressure decreases proportionately as atmospheric pressure (expressed as barometric pressure) decreases.

Your body is affected by the pressure of gases surrounding it. Thus, as you ascend, the percentage of each gas in the atmosphere remains the same but remember that there are fewer molecules at less pressure that your body can use (or eliminate). The lack of O_2, for example, at a pressure necessary to carry it to your blood cells, is what leads to hypoxia.

Henry's Law states that the amount of gas in solution, not chemically combined, varies directly with the partial pressure of that gas over the solution. Thus, when the pressure of a gas over a certain liquid decreases, the amount of that gas dissolved in the liquid also decreases (and vice versa). When equilibrium is reached, the dissolved gas pressure equals the partial pressure of the gas in the atmosphere to which a solution is exposed. Thus, as the pressure falls, as during ascent, the amount of gas that can be held in solution is reduced. Open a bottle of pop. Watch the sudden release of bubbles as the bottle pressure equals ambient pressure. This occurs as a result of Henry's Law (Fig. 1-3).

The same thing can happen in your body. There are additional factors that influence and modify the process of gas uptake and elimination, such as the varying types of fluids in your body, the circulation rate and volume of your blood, and the amount of hemoglobin (Hgb) in your blood, among others.

Graham's Law states that a gas of high pressure exerts a force toward a region of lower pressure, and that if an existing permeable membrane separates these regions of unequal pressure, the gas of higher pressure will pass (or diffuse) through the membrane into the region of lower pressure. For example, this law explains the transfer of oxygen from one part of your body

Fig. 1-3 The amount of gas dissolved in solution is directly proportional to the pressure of the gas over the solution.

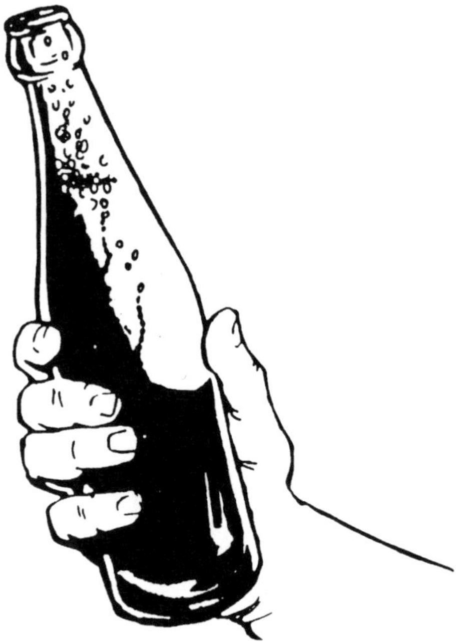

to another as it passes through your blood vessel walls and also in your lung's breathing tubes. Each gas behaves independently of the other gases in solution and therefore may move in opposite directions to another gas of differing partial pressure. This sounds confusing but what is important to keep in mind is that oxygen in solution in the blood, for example, can pass across or through your body's membranes to reach other tissues.

How the Atmosphere Affects You

In addition to the pressure and temperature divisions of the atmosphere, the atmosphere also can be divided into zones that affect you medically and physiologically. When you are flying, be suspicious of any performance that is not considered acceptable to you or your crewmate because it could be the result of hypoxia or other conditions directly related to the content of the air surrounding you, even in a pressurized cabin.

The physiological efficient zone extends from sea level to about 10,000 to 12,000 feet and is where your body is adapted or can become adapted to detrimental atmospheric changes. The barometric pressure drops by almost 300 mm of Hg. The O_2 amounts (not percentages) are usually sufficient to maintain acceptable performance without supplemental oxygen—if you are healthy. Rapid changes after prolonged time at any altitude, however, can result in a situation that could be incapacitating, such as experiencing ear blocks. Decompression sickness (or bends) is rare in this zone.

In the physiological deficient zone, you have an increased risk of developing problems, especially hypoxia, trapped gas, and evolved gas situations (the bends). This deficient zone extends from the top of the physiological efficient zone to about 50,000 feet. You cannot exist above this altitude unless you are in a pressurized suit or cabin. Therefore, your body responds as if you were in deep space.

By understanding this hostile environment, you can respect your working conditions, rather than just assuming that it's "dangerous up there" because someone said so; you can reason for yourself what the risks really are and anticipate potential problems. Ear blocks and hypoxia are common. Yet, as long as you feel Okay, you are often not aware of a potential problem simply because you are not suspecting anything. How you feel is often a poor predictor of being safe.

Despite war stories of pilots pressing on through the elements at all altitudes without supplemental O_2, your body still is affected by conditions related to traditional gas laws—hypoxia, bends, ear blocks, and other subtle conditions. Therefore, if you are in the atmosphere anywhere above the level in which you live, you are at risk, no matter how you perceive your performance. Simply being in flight invites potential and often undetected changes in your piloting skills. Flying at any altitude is safe and well tolerated if you are knowledgeable and protected, but the atmosphere is not forgiving if its physical properties are taken for granted.

How You Are Constructed

In this section, I briefly discuss each major anatomical system: brain, musculoskeletal, gastrointestinal, metabolic, and circulatory. Knowledge of these systems provides you with some insight into how the body should work under ideal and controllable situations. More importantly, it should raise your level of awareness of what can happen in less-than-ideal conditions. Then, and only then, can you take corrective action to either avoid unsafe situations or to be prepared to cope with the physiological and psychological challenges of flight.

When considering the abnormal body, we usually think of *pathology*, which is the medical term referring to anything that is not normal. One frequent form of pathology of any part of the body is an inflammation of that part. Inflammation can result either from an infection or from an irritation or injury. Every part of your body can be potentially inflamed. It is inflammation if the name of a body part ends in *-itis*. Thus, when you hear such terms as tendonitis, tonsillitis, appendicitis, arthritis (*arthro*, meaning joint), meningitis (*menin,* meaning covering of the brain), carditis (*cardi*, meaning heart), and so on, you are talking about an inflammation. The intensity of the inflammation determines your level of impairment.

Let's talk about how your body is supposed to work when it is on the ground.

Your Body's Electrical System

The brain is the most important part of your total nervous system, also called your central nervous system (CNS). It controls all functions, physiological, mechanical, and mental, by sending electrical and chemical signals to the various parts of your body, much like a computer. Instead of using wires, your brain transmits a signal via nerve cells. A row of these cells is called a *nerve,* often extending from the brain, through the spinal cord, and to one of your body parts.

As explained previously, various parts of your brain can become infected or inflamed such as occurs with meningitis and encephalitis. The same is true of injury. Because your brain is in a closed container (the skull), any impact to the skull can tear blood vessels, bruise brain cells, or cause swelling of your brain. A descriptive analogy to explaining a closed head injury is to consider what happens to a fresh tomato that just fits inside a jar. Drop the jar. The tomato bounces back and forth (a rebound effect) within the jar with expected results—a softer tomato. Therefore, any closed head injury could represent injury to the brain and requires extensive evaluation and treatment to determine the degree of injury.

A *concussion*, by definition, is any period of unconsciousness. If you experience loss of consciousness (LOC) for any reason, the potential for brain damage exists. Brain damage puts you at potential risk for other problems, especially in flight, that may range from a simple headache to convulsions, at unpredictable times. Hypoxia is known to trigger unpredictable, serious symptoms in anyone with a history of brain pathology. Therefore, any brain pathology is a potential risk to safe flying until it can be medically proven that the risk is acceptable.

The spinal cord is an extension of your brain, like a bundle of wires. Signals from the various parts of your brain are transmitted to the rest of your body by this cable of nerves. In addition, it brings back signals from your body parts in a form of feedback that the brain then processes with other information needed to function. For example, your brain tells you to turn the ignition on with your fingers. When the sound of the engine reaches your ear, that signal is transmitted back to your brain to tell you to release the ignition switch. All these signals pass through your spinal cord.

Any pathology in your spinal cord interferes with proper information flow to and from your brain. Any injury to your spinal cord results in total loss of neurological control to your body parts. Any nerve can be infected and inflamed.

The peripheral nervous system is an extension of your spinal cord. The signals to and from your brain are transmitted to the various organs and parts of your body via a series of smaller, single nerves in your peripheral nervous system. It's like a telephone trunk line coming into your house and then branching off into your extension phones in different rooms. Each muscle and organ cell has one or more nerves controlling its functions.

Control of your body functions is more complex than just a

single nerve telling an organ or body part what to do. Many functions are automatic; that is, they do not require a conscious effort on your part to initiate action. Such processes are controlled by the autonomic or sympathetic nervous system, and include breathing, digestion, heart rate, blood pressure, internal temperature control, and many more activities. The feedback from your various organs, like a home temperature thermostat, tells your brain what it needs and then your brain responds without your intervention.

This is what happens in a fight-or-flight situation. When you are suddenly alarmed, scared, facing a dangerous activity, or other situation requiring a quick response, your brain senses the urgency and, in addition to sending electrical signals, also releases chemicals and hormones (commonly adrenaline). All of these situations increase your body's metabolism so you can respond to the emergency. Often this response is instantaneous. Everyone has experienced a rush of adrenaline: the rapid heart rate, tingling sensation, and other symptoms in a dangerous situation. Remember that near-hit while driving in your car or the feeling when your doctor says your blood pressure is high?

Control of our senses is also automatic. You see, hear, taste, smell, and feel without having to consciously ask the brain to act. Your brain is always on, and you are continuously receiving cues from your sense organs, especially your ears, nose, and skin. And it's automatic. Pain is a good example. You can reach for a hot pan on the stove, and pick it up through conscious commands. If it's too hot you automatically—instinctively—let go and pull your hand back, probably dropping the pan. This happens so quickly that you are usually unable to intercede before dropping the pan and consciously hang on. What you do next requires a conscious effort. Do you leave the pan alone, pick it up with oven gloves, or throw water on it?

You can learn to hold onto the hot pan even if is hot. This is a trained response. The same holds true in flying. Many actions and functions of flight are contrary to what your body thinks it ought to do without your input. It is very important to be familiar with flight conditions that are not usually well tolerated by your body.

Your Human Airframe

Bones, tendons, ligaments, and muscles—they all hold your body together and encase the organs that allow you to function. They make up the musculoskeletal system that packages your components and allows you to participate in life's activities. Most of these parts are used in some way in some part of flight. Others, obviously, are not essential to fly. Given the appropriate tools and controls, and the proof of performance through trial and error, many people can fly without a perfect body.

The covering, or skin, is actually another body organ. In fact, it's the largest in your body. Your skull houses the brain and most of your sense organs—nose, ears, eyes, and tongue. Your chest contains the lungs and heart, and the pelvis protects the abdomen and supports the body by being attached to your legs. The rest of your bones are used to manipulate your body and perform a variety of functions (walking, sitting, picking up things, and flying airplanes if you're a pilot).

Your skeletal parts require joints to move. Most joints are like simple hinges; others, like your hips' and shoulders' ball-and-socket joints have a wide range of motion. All joints are held together with ligaments. Tendons are the links between your moving bones and your muscles. One end of the muscle is attached directly to the bone and the other end uses the tendon to attach to a variety of locations on the bone. Muscles can do only one thing—contract—and this contraction bends the joint. Muscle contraction is an activity that requires energy, generates heat, and displays various levels of strength.

You are born with the same amount of muscle tissue that you have now. You do not add muscles when you exercise, but you can increase the size of each muscle cell. The effectiveness of a muscle group is dependent on your physical condition and whether or not your muscles and tissues are getting adequate oxygen and nutrients. Therefore, exercise and a balanced diet are important for more reasons than keeping you looking good and protecting your heart.

Injuries are the most common pathology to your musculoskeletal system. Your body is remarkably capable of rebuilding these tissues if you allow time to heal and protect the part from further injury or aggravation. Often, a pilot tends to get anxious and puts an injured part back to work only to be re-injured. Inflammation is another very common problem. Tendonitis, arthritis, and myositis are the usual results. Tendons and ligaments are particularly slow to heal because of their low blood supply. In contrast, muscles have a large blood supply and heal fairly quickly. Muscles, therefore, are easily bruised (a bruise is bleeding into your muscle tissues and under your skin).

Your Working Parts

The purpose of your gastrointestinal (GI) system, or tract, is to provide and digest nutrients and fluids for metabolism into tissue cells. Fortunately, eating remains one of the pleasures of life and we often make excess of that pleasure. Foods and fluids that you ingest are transformed into energy, tissue rebuilding, and maintenance of bodily functions.

Your GI tract is essentially one long tube beginning at your mouth and ending at the anus. Fluids are quickly absorbed through the walls of the GI tract and transferred to your bloodstream. The first part of digestion is that food is physically broken up with chewing, then converted into basic components (mostly glucose and amino acids) in the rest of your GI tract. All waste products (indigestible components and metabolic byproducts) are passed out of the body through your large intestine.

Fluids are absorbed and excreted throughout this whole process. The absorbed fluids replace those lost through metabolism, sweating, and urination.

In your large intestine (colon and cecum), undigestible material is collected, compacted, and then further broken down by bacteria. This bacterial action often generates gas that can be passed out of body orifices. As this material, now called fecal matter, continues down the large intestine, fluids are again exchanged to maintain a soft consistency. Constipation results if there are not enough undigested fibers to absorb water. A bowel movement allows this material to pass from the large intestine, through the rectum, and out the anus.

Digestion is a circadian rhythm. Thus, an internal rhythm tells your body when to expect food. This triggers hunger and stimulates your digestive fluids. Peristalsis (the contractions of the bowel to assist movement of food through the GI tract) also begins. Digestion at odd times may be inefficient if food intake is out of synchrony with your physiological rhythms.

Within the GI tract, the most common problems are intestinal flus, inflammation (gastritis), constipation, and hemorrhoids, all of minimal concern. Ulcers, bleeding ulcers, and tumors are of major concern.

Your metabolic system is what makes all your organs and musculoskeletal system work. Your nervous system supplies the information and direction, your musculoskeletal system is the container and does the mechanical work, your GI system processes the fuel and building material, and your metabolic system converts these resources into substances, chemicals, energy, etc., all of which support the activities of the body.

Your liver is located in the upper right hand corner of your abdomen, partially under your rib cage, and is the organ carrying most of the metabolic workload for your body. This organ (sometimes called a chemical processing plant) plays an essential role of metabolism. It makes glycogen (the body's storage form of glucose), processes fats and proteins, removes waste products, and generates heat for the body.

The liver is important in changing the simple chemicals absorbed from the GI tract into usable products. These products

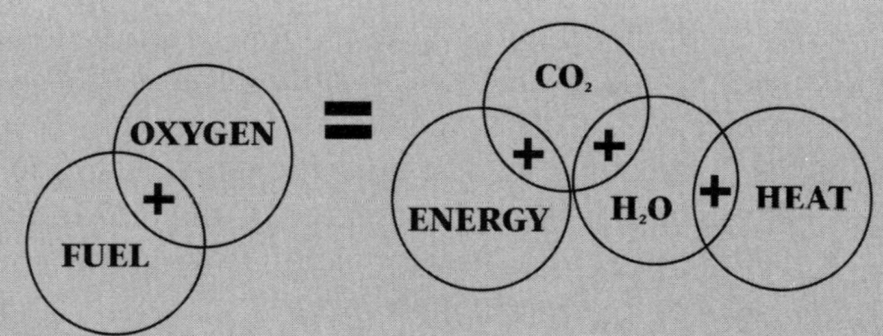

Metabolism: Some of the chemical and physical processes that maintain life.

include vitamins, enzymes, bile, and cholesterol. In addition, it detoxifies drugs, medications, and alcohol.

Your gallbladder, which is like a small bag, stores bile made by the liver. It also can form "stones" that can block the tube to the intestine and keep the bile from entering the GI tract. This backup can interfere with hepatic (liver) function.

From a metabolic point of view, alcohol is a toxin to the liver. As a result, there is often an increased production of certain enzymes used to detoxify alcohol. These enzymes can be measured in blood tests, indicating that the liver is being affected.

Your kidneys (located on both sides of the spine just below the back of the rib cage) filter your blood. They take out impurities and some waste products. An important function of your kidneys is to maintain fluid balance in the body. The kidneys, therefore, adjust the volume of blood in your circulatory system by conserving or excreting water. Furthermore, they adjust the composition of the blood to ensure the right balance of essential products. If there is not enough fluid (water) as serum within the blood, the kidneys conserve water by concentrating your urine. Concentrated urine is dark yellow compared with pale yellow, indicating adequate hydration.

Because your kidneys are capable of regulating urine concentration, you can rarely drink too much water. There is certainly a major problem of too little fluids. In fact, dehydration is a real concern and results in prolonged concentrated urine.

A problem relatively common in aviation is kidney stones. Concentrated urine from dehydration over many months tends to form small sand-sized "stones." If small enough, they pass out of your body without producing any symptoms. If a stone gets stuck in the ureter or at the entrance to the bladder, however, severe pain can suddenly result. Some people are prone to making kidney stones. Therefore, once one stone is made, such a person is at higher risk of making others. It is essential in preventing stone formation to maintain a high level of hydration, especially on long trips.

The pancreas is located to the left of the liver. Its primary function is to produce insulin. All body tissues require insulin for metabolism of glucose into energy. At certain times of the day, the pancreas is programmed to begin producing insulin.

Thus, there is a circadian component that has a bearing on becoming hypoglycemic, a topic to be discussed later.

Diabetes is a disease in which there is not enough insulin produced or none at all. Insulin-dependent diabetics need to inject insulin into their bodies to maintain a balanced availability for use in metabolizing glucose. Some diabetics can make a little insulin but they need the help of an oral medication. This is a chemical (not an oral insulin) that stimulates the pancreas to make and secrete more insulin plus makes cells use insulin more efficiently. Diet becomes a special concern in maintaining a proper insulin level because the pancreas is stimulated by the presence or absence of some key foods (such as sugars, carbohydrates, and fats).

Your thyroid is a gland located at the front of your lower neck, right in the middle. It makes two different hormones each of which plays a significant role in establishing metabolic rate or the speed with which your body functions and responds to activities. Too high of a rate makes you hyperactive, resulting in weight loss, nervousness, and a sense of warmth. The other hormone assists in the metabolism of calcium and bones.

Your Hydraulic System

As I just discussed, your metabolic system is critical to making your body work. It is the circulatory system, however, that provides the mechanism for the transfer of energy and nutrients for metabolism. It transports your blood, which in turn carries essential O_2, nutrients, and waste products. This system includes fluid (blood), a pump (heart), tubing (blood vessels), and your body parts (organs) that require support of the circulation system. Therefore, it is comparable to any closed hydraulic system in your airplane. It is this system that is of most interest to you because any change in O_2 levels immediately changes the performance of many organs, especially the brain.

The heart is the pump in this human hydraulic system. It is a closed structure with blood flowing from your heart, into arteries, then through capillaries that are spread around the tissues. From there, your blood continues into the venous system, and back to the heart.

Your heart pump is divided into four chambers that take blood from a major vein and pump it into arteries (Fig. 1-4). The two smaller chambers on top (the atria) take in blood from the veins and pump it into the larger ventricles below. The ventricles then pump blood to the lungs and to the rest of your body. The heart is muscle and responds just like any other muscle in your body. Every muscle fiber must contract at the same time to function properly, and these contractions squeeze blood through the one-way heart valves. The blood moves forward but not backward so there is a moment when blood pressure goes down during this transition between contractions.

Also, like any other muscle, your heart needs a blood supply. Blood is supplied via the coronary arteries. It is these arteries that become blocked in heart disease, sometimes leading to heart attacks or poor blood profusion of the heart muscles (called ischemia). Oxygen needs to get to your heart muscle for energy. If it doesn't, the heart can fail or become less effective in pumping blood throughout your body. Total blockage of blood to your heart muscle leads to death of some of the tissues

Fig. 1-4 The heart is the pump of the circulatory system.

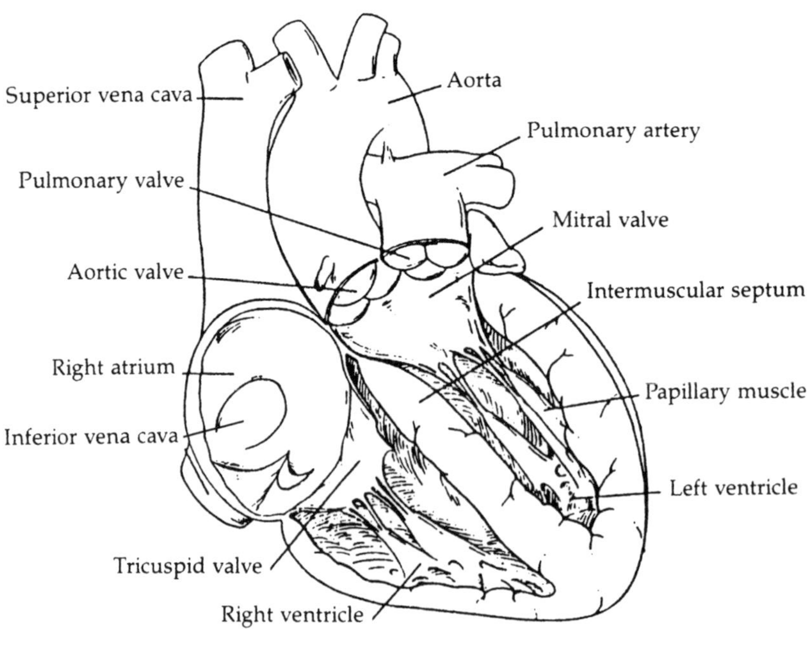

of your heart. Dead heart tissue is called a myocardial infarction (*myo,* meaning muscle; *cardia*, meaning heart; *infarction*, meaning dead), or MI. This is another name for heart attack.

If your heart muscle fibers do not contract simultaneously, changes occur in the rhythm and contractility. Fibrillation occurs when your muscle fibers are contracting at different times and not together. Looking at heart muscles in fibrillation is like looking at a can of live worms, each one trying to do its own thing. Any of these rhythm problems leads to heart failure or an inefficient pump.

The amount of blood that flows out of your heart per any period of time is dependent on several conditions: the heart rate (pulse), the volume of blood ejected from the heart, and the force of the contraction. Much of these activities are controlled by the autonomic nervous system, thus, you don't consciously have to tell the heart to function.

In your lungs, O_2 and CO_2 are exchanged from the ambient air with that in the blood. This exchange takes place in the alveoli (Fig. 1-5). Your lungs are structured like an upside-down tree. Air enters the lungs through your mouth or nose, passes into your pharynx and trachea, and then goes to the main bronchus. This large breathing tube then splits into two bronchi that further split into thousands of smaller bronchioles or miniature breathing tubes. Therefore, all air inhaled

Risk Factors for Coronary Heart Disease

- Gender (especially males)
- Family history of premature heart disease
- Cigarette smoking
- Low HDL(<35 mg/dL)
- High total cholesterol (>200)
- High LDL (>150)
- Diabetes mellitus
- Hypertension
- Severe obesity (>30% overweight)
- Presence of arteriosclerosis
- Sedentary lifestyle
- Low fiber intake

Fig. 1-5 The lung resembles an upside-down tree.

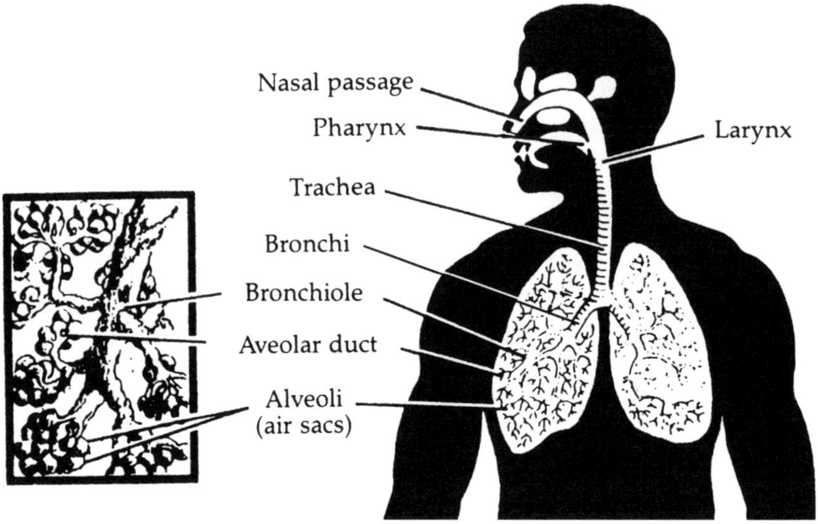

ends up in tiny alveoli (tiny rubberlike balloons). Capillaries (miniature blood vessels) surround these alveoli and, because their walls are so thin, gases can pass (diffuse) back and forth. Blood in these capillaries accesses the gases through diffusion.

Air is pulled into your lungs by decreasing the pressure within your chest cavity. The diaphragm is a muscular dome-shaped floor of the lower part of the rib cage that forms a closed container with only one opening—the bronchial tree. When this muscle contracts, it flattens out, creating lower pressure, and allowing air to fill the alveoli. Inhalation from contractions of the diaphragm is an active process. Exhaling is passive because the diaphragm relaxes and returns to its dome shape. The muscles between your ribs enhance this activity. Respiration is also an autonomic function, just like your heart rate. It is controlled by your brain. With exercise, both breathing and heart rate are increased without you having to think about them.

The hydraulic link between your heart, lungs, brain, and other body parts is the blood vessels (Fig. 1-6). Arteries carry O_2-rich blood from the lungs to the tissues and are unique from veins in that they have muscle and elastic cells within their walls. This structure allows them to dilate or constrict, an effective way of increasing or decreasing blood flow to various parts of your body. For example, while running, your leg muscles need more blood. Arteries to these muscles automatically dilate to their full size, permitting a larger volume of blood to reach the tissues. The same process controls your body temperatures.

Fig. 1-6 Essential oxygen and nutrients are transported throughout the body by the circulatory system.

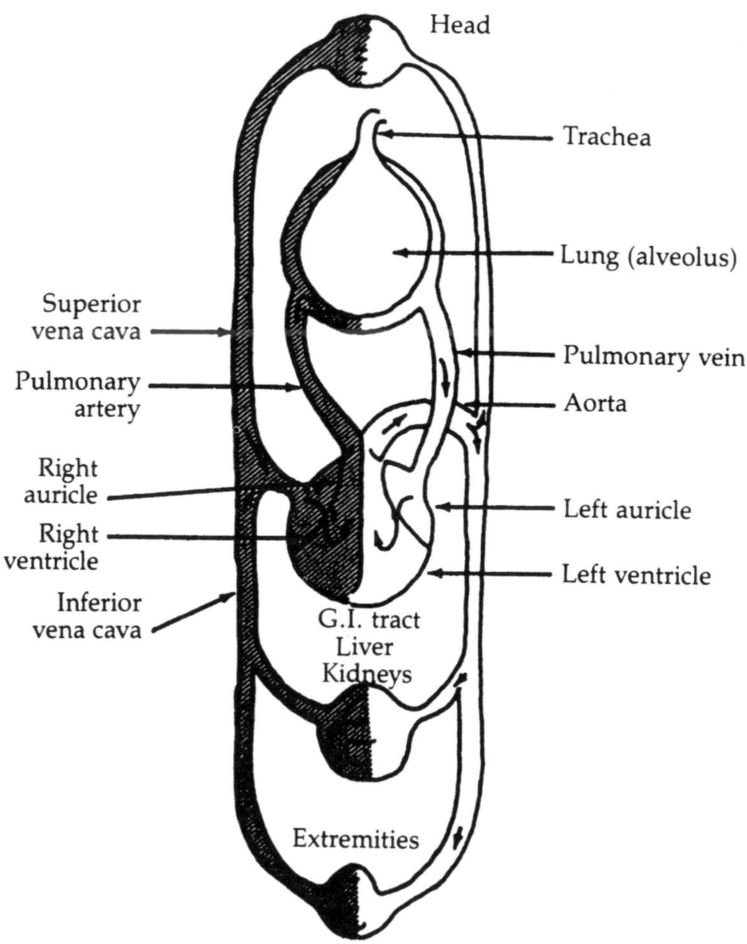

The elasticity of arterial walls helps to keep your blood pressure constant during the relaxed period between heart contractions. The pressure within the artery resulting from this elasticity enhances and prolongs the pressure that is generated by the heart—like blowing up a balloon.

Veins are simple tubes without muscles or elastic tissues. Veins carry blood that is deficient in O_2. Some veins in your arms and legs prevent blood from flowing backward during the relaxation period. This can happen because they have one-way valves scattered throughout the length of the vein.

Blood pressure within your veins is very low. Muscles, such as those in your legs, surround the veins. When the muscles contract, they compress the vessel's wall and "milk" the blood forward to the heart. This is often called the "muscle pump." Blood can pool in the extremities when sitting for long periods of time, resulting in stagnant hypoxia.

Respiration is the exchange of gases between your body tissues and the ambient air. The main objective is to add O_2 and remove CO_2. About 90 percent of blood is water (serum). Part of the nonserum blood is a red blood cell that physically carries O_2 molecules attached to a chemical on the cell called

Fig. 1-7 Arterial and venous blood saturation for normal sea level conditions.

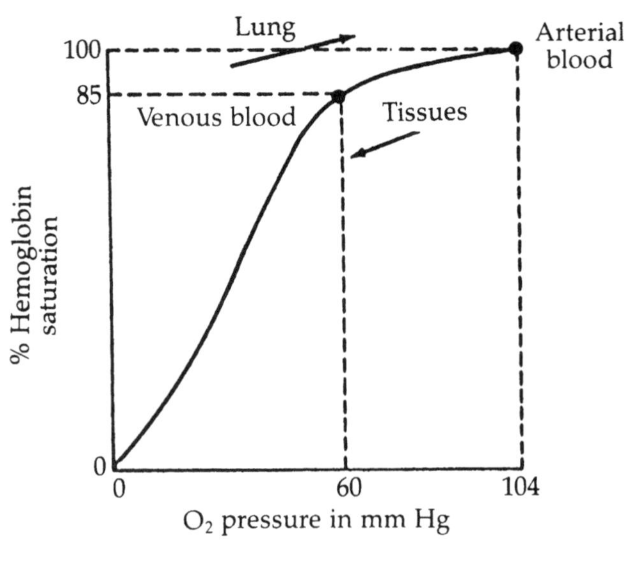

hemoglobin. The red blood cells become the transporters of O_2 by using hemoglobin. Any change in the hemoglobin, number of red blood cells, or diffusion of gases causes some form of hypoxia.

The dark color of venous blood is an indication of hemoglobin that has no O_2 attached. The bright red color of arterial blood results from the combination of O_2 with hemoglobin. The amount of O_2 carried by the red blood cells is normally about 95 to 98 percent of saturation of the cell. This is called the *oxygen dissociation curve* and indicates that available O_2 falls rapidly when the saturation goes below 90 percent (Fig. 1-7) and hypoxia develops.

Gases move across the vascular membranes by the process of diffusion. Because of the physics of gases, a gas can move from an area of high pressure to an area of lower pressure. The same process of diffusion occurs at the tissue and cellular levels within your body.

Obviously, your body is far more complex than what is described herein. To understand how the physiology of flight can affect your performance, however, you must have a basic understanding of how the body works. Furthermore, anything that interferes with a normally functioning body, such as the status of your health, also can determine if you can pass Federal Aviation Administration (FAA) medical standards.

Flying above 5,000 feet AGL 2

Judy and her family left Des Moines for a skiing weekend in Colorado. Their single-engine Piper performed flawlessly and they landed uneventfully at the Vail airport, in time for some late-afternoon skiing. They felt tired but attributed that to the long, hard workweek and to the flight. After 2 days of skiing, they headed home, except now they were very fatigued and Judy found it difficult to concentrate and to focus, even though she was never above 5,000 feet AGL (above ground level). A nagging headache and general lethargy persisted. As the airplane continued on to Des Moines, she was able to get her aircraft below 5,000 feet MSL (mean sea level) and she began to feel better. Although she was uncomfortable during the beginning of the flight, she also recognized that she was hypoxic from several days at an altitude to which her body was not accustomed. She left her O_2 mask on for several minutes after getting to a lower altitude. Had she not suspected hypoxia, she would have been even more impaired.

WHEN SOMEONE TALKS to you about high-altitude physiology, they are commonly referring to conditions that affect your body as a result of being at an altitude where airliners fly. They think that you should be concerned about hypoxia, ear blocks, etc., only at these high (whatever high means) altitudes. In actuality, however, anytime you remain at an altitude above which you are accustomed, there is a risk of problems developing. Therefore, the information in this chapter is not only for airline pilots flying above 18,000 feet but also for pilots or flight attendants flying at any altitude, which would include recreational flying, helicopter activities, and low-level commercial flights.

Hypoxia, trapped gas situations, and decompression sickness—often called the *bends*—are the most common problems directly related to the physical properties of the different layers of the atmosphere. In addition, scuba diving has become very popular and complicates your decision to fly because the physiological effects of a dive may linger long after the dive is over. It is therefore essential for you to be able to identify the symptoms of any of these conditions, either in yourself or in your crewmate. As a responsible pilot or flight attendant, you should maintain a high index of suspicion for potential high-altitude problems and respond with immediate and appropriate action before an ear block or hypoxia occurs.

Essential Oxygen

The lack of adequate O_2 in your body's metabolism is called *hypoxia* (or *anoxia* for the total absence of O_2). It is this lack of sufficient O_2 to your body's tissues and cells that can impair you in flight. This situation occurs for reasons in addition to the reduced availability of O_2 in the air you breath, such as your blood's ability to carry O_2, and the interference of drugs, alcohol, carbon monoxide, smoking, and illness, to name a few. Many incidents and some accidents are officially related to a pilot's inability to detect that he or she was hypoxic, even mildly so. Such a pilot's performance becomes unsafe because of compromised skills and judgment, pilot error, and lack of respect or understanding of hypoxia and its affects. To fully understand the challenge in getting O_2 to your cells, you must understand the physiology of O_2. Then you can understand and respect hypoxia, no matter what the cause.

Classification of Hypoxia

No matter why you are hypoxic, the symptoms and effects on your flying skills are basically the same. The following classification is therefore intended only to review potential *causes* so that your degree of suspicion about being hypoxic (or observing hypoxia in crew or passengers) is raised, especially when you are flying under situations that put you at higher risk.

Hypoxic (Altitude) Hypoxia

Hypoxic hypoxia is the most common kind of hypoxia. It is, however, only one of four kinds. It is associated with lack of

HYPOXIA

SYMPTOMS (Subjective)

- Air hunger
- Apprehension
- Fatigue
- Nausea
- Headache
- Dizziness
- Hot and cold flashes
- Euphoria
- Belligerence
- Blurred vision
- Tunnel vision
- Numbness
- Tingling

SIGNS (Objective)

- Hyperventilation
- Cyanosis
- Mental confusion
- Poor judgment
- Muscle incoordination

→ **UNCONSCIOUSNESS** ←

available O_2 in the air you breathe, such as experienced when flying at altitude in an unpressurized cabin. In hypoxic hypoxia, there isn't enough O_2 available to bring into your lungs with sufficient partial pressure; this situation can occur as you ascend. The number of molecules of O_2 decreases, although the percentage of O_2 in the air remains the same. Hypoxic hypoxia is particularly evident in the physiologically deficient zone of the atmosphere. Strictly speaking, you are hypoxic even at a few thousand feet above the ground. In actuality, the symptoms do not become significant until about 5,000 feet, especially at night. The significance and impact of the symptoms on your performance are related to many factors, which are explained later. Regardless, hypoxia should be a concern at all altitudes.

According to the gas laws, hypoxic hypoxia exists when the partial pressure of O_2 in the atmosphere and the inhaled ambient air is reduced as it travels into your bronchial tree and into the lungs. Thus, the partial pressure of O_2 as it is made available to your blood within the lungs is too low to effectively transfer enough O_2 to the blood and then to the cells of your body tissues.

Hypemic (Anemic) Hypoxia

Hypemic hypoxia occurs when the blood's ability to carry or transport O_2 is compromised, even though there is adequate O_2 available to breathe. There are a variety of reasons for this condition to occur. Anemia, or the reduced number of healthy, functioning red blood cells for any reason (disease, blood loss, deformed blood cells, etc.) results in a lowered capacity for blood to carry O_2. Hemoglobin (Hgb), a chemical part of the red blood cell, physically and chemically carries (by combining with O_2) more O_2 molecules than are dissolved in solution in the serum. Anything that interferes or displaces the O_2 that is attached to the Hgb thus reduces the amount of O_2 carried to the cell. A lowered O_2-carrying capacity occurs most commonly when CO is inhaled. CO attaches to the Hgb displacing O_2. Other chemicals cause the same combining interference on Hgb, such as sulfa drugs and nitrites found in food preservatives.

Stagnant Hypoxia

If the blood flow (the circulation of the O_2-carrying Hgb in red blood cells) is compromised for any reason, then sufficient O_2 cannot physically reach your cells and tissues. Stagnant implies a diminished flow, not necessarily complete shutdown. Such a decrease in blood flow results from the heart failing to pump effectively, an artery constricting and cutting off the flow, and venous pooling of blood such as in varicose veins of the legs. Sitting for long periods of time tends to enhance this pooling. Another cause, unique to flying, is "positive G" maneuvers—pulling Gs—and long periods of pressure breathing at extreme cabin altitudes where O_2 masks are required. Another situation is in cold temperatures where your blood supply to your extremities is decreased.

Histotoxic Hypoxia

Histotoxic means that the cell expecting and needing O_2 is abnormal or unable to accept the O_2. Thus, the O_2 may be inhaled or reach tissues or cells in adequate amounts, but it is unable to be used and metabolized once it is there. This can occur when alcohol is present in the blood or in the cells. Alcohol becomes, in effect, a toxin to these cells. The same is true for some narcotics and certain poisons, such as cyanide.

Stages of Hypoxia

A lack of O_2 (hypoxia) results in a variety of subtle and not-so-subtle symptoms, no matter what the reason is for O_2 not getting into or being used by cells. The danger of hypoxia is that you probably are unsuspecting when you are hypoxic. The key to flying safe at altitude is to first recognize the conditions under which you could become hypoxic. Then,the symptoms you know are your individual indicators for being hypoxic must be respected by you. Equally important, you must be able to recognize hypoxia in a crewmate.

Most hypoxic symptoms are related, directly or indirectly, to the nervous system because the tissues of your nervous system have a profound requirement for O_2, especially the brain (and eyes). If hypoxia is prolonged, serious problems develop progressively and could ultimately lead to death. In extreme cases (prior to death), some brain cells are actually killed and they cannot be regenerated (Fig. 2-1).

It bears repeating that because hypoxia can be, and often is, gradual in its development, you must recognize its various

Fig. 2-1 Stages of hypoxia.

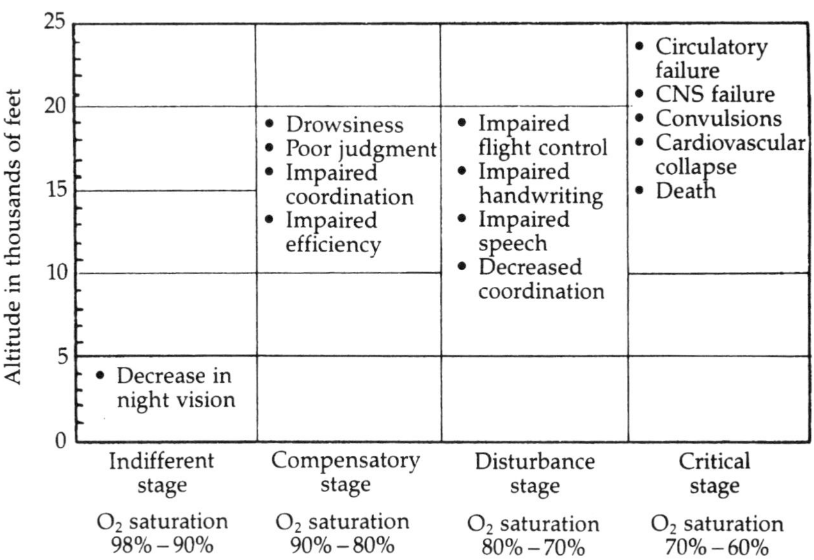

stages, especially in yourself. If symptoms in the early stages are identified, assume you are hypoxic. The earlier hypoxia can be recognized, the sooner corrective action can be taken before you mentally become unable to act appropriately by donning your O_2 mask.

Keep in mind that, although altitude is the common denominator in being hypoxic, your health can affect your tolerance to the conditions leading to hypoxia. Other abuses such as smoking, alcohol, and stress can reduce tolerance even if you are healthy. Therefore, hypoxia can be very unpredictable for you or your crewmates. Experiencing no problem at 10,000 feet last week does not mean that you will be safe from hypoxia again at the same altitude.

Indifferent Stage

One of the earliest symptoms of hypoxia is its affect on your eyes because the eyes are anatomically an extension of the brain. Therefore, vision, especially your night vision, can deteriorate even at altitudes less than 5,000 feet AGL. And you won't know you are having problems because you can't compare what you are actually seeing with what you should be seeing. For example, night vision is lost by 5 to 10 percent at 5,000 feet, 15 to 25 percent at 10,000 feet, and 25 to 30 percent at 12,000 feet. Other classical symptoms, in addition to impaired vision, can be present at lower altitudes if your body is not tolerant, as will be explained later. Regardless, when you are flying at any altitude at night, be aware that your vision and other mental skills may be compromised.

Compensatory Stage

During the compensatory stage, your body and mind are quickly approaching the point where they can be severely affected and in increasingly subtle ways. Your circulatory system and, to a lesser degree, your respiratory system can provide some defense against hypoxia in this stage. As a result of increased heart rate, enhanced circulation, and a more productive heart pumping blood, you can still cope. Respiration (breathing rate and depth) also increases. Although these responses are automatic, you should not assume you are recovering without taking immediate, conscious corrective action whenever you suspect hypoxia.

At 12,000 to 15,000 feet the effects of hypoxia on the nervous system may become increasingly incapacitating, especially if you are unacclimated. As the amount of time at this altitude increases (as little as 10 to 15 minutes), impairment of skills becomes very evident, especially as observed by others. A variety of symptoms develop, many of which compromise your flying performance and skill. These symptoms include drowsiness, poor judgment, and frequent subtle errors in flying skills. A more dangerous manifestation to you is a feeling of well-being and indifference (euphoria). Once again, the crucial characteristic about hypoxia, especially in this stage, is your recognition of an increasing O_2 deficit before you become unaware that you are in trouble.

Disturbance Stage

During the disturbance stage, your probability of recovery is greatly diminished because you missed your chance to intervene. Symptoms become more severe with headache, hyperventilation, impaired peripheral vision, marked fatigue, and sleepiness common. And especially euphoria. By now you might even recognize that you are hypoxic, but you don't care and have little incentive to take a corrective action, such as getting to a lower altitude or going on O_2. You may actually be unable to physically reach for the O_2 mask and put it on, although mentally realizing that you should be doing something.

Critical Stage

The critical stage is when you have lost it—you're unconscious. All this can happen within 3 to 5 minutes after you failed to recognize you were hypoxic during the compensatory and disturbance stages. Some pilots faint as a result of circulatory failure or improper functioning of the central nervous system.

Symptoms of Hypoxia

The following are some of the more common symptoms experienced by hypoxic pilots.

- Change in peripheral vision, even noting tunnel vision.
- Visual acuity impairment, images appear slightly blurred, can't focus.

- Difficulty in visual accommodation or focusing from near to distant objects.
- Weakness in muscles, it's more difficult to change the airplane seat.
- Feeling very tired and fatigued, sleepy for no reason (not due to boredom).
- Headache, especially if hypoxic for a long period (2 or more hours).
- Light-headedness and mild dizziness, you react poorly in tight turns.
- Tingling in fingers and toes.
- Muscular coordination decreased, you're sloppy at controls.
- Stammering, can't get the right words out to ATC.
- Impaired judgment, doing dumb things, slow thinking.
- Altered respiration, breathing faster and shallower.
- Reaction time decreased, you've lost your touch in flying.
- Greatly reduced night vision (even at 5,000 feet).
- Euphoria.

Many of these symptoms are subjective; that is, most are not definitive of your level of hypoxia. For example, a change in heart rate is objective evidence but it also can change with exertion, stress, and other physical situations. You may not think of being hypoxic. A common symptom is fatigue, another very subjective sign of hypoxia. How fatigued must you be for you to suspect hypoxia? Are you fatigued from hypoxia or from the length of the flight? And if you are indeed hypoxic, you may be complacent about any degree of fatigue. Also, these symptoms are not listed in order of importance or ease of recognition. Some pilots experience a specific kind of headache, whereas others only recollect being fatigued or uncoordinated before they become incapacitated and lose control.

Hypoxia is common and it happens to all pilots and flight attendants, many times, in varying degrees. It is unfortunate that the human body does not have an effective warning system to alert you to the onset of hypoxia. Hypoxia is painless. Each pilot reacts differently to the same degree of hypoxia and he or she experiences different symptoms and impairments. These individual symptoms also can change as you get older. It is for these reasons that the military continues to periodically expose its flight crews to an altitude chamber ride. This ride allows a pilot to experience what his or her symptoms are for hypoxia before reaching the disturbance stage wherein one cannot (or will not) recover or take appropriate action. No amount of lecturing or reading prepares you for how you detect your own level of incapacitating hypoxia, let alone respect its impact on your performance. Therefore, it is strongly encouraged that, at least once in your flying life, you take an altitude chamber ride.

In summary, the signs and symptoms of hypoxia are many and varied, they differ from individual to individual, and are unpredictable at any given time and altitude. Be aware, be suspicious, and watch your crewmate!

Factors Influencing Your Tolerance to Hypoxia

As mentioned, it is impossible to predict exactly when, where, or how hypoxic reactions will occur in you because individuals vary widely in their susceptibility to O_2 deficiency. This susceptibility is related to many factors that you can control. Avoidance of these factors becomes part of your responsibility to preclude unexpected hypoxia symptoms.

Self-Imposed Factors

Although the cabin may be at less than 10,000 feet (pressure altitude), your body reacts as though it is at physiological altitude. The following self-imposed factors raise this physiological altitude, and your mind and body react accordingly with some degree of incapacitation. So, for example, instead of your body performing at a 10,000-foot altitude, it responds as if it were at 13,000 feet.

Alcohol

Alcohol in your body can result in histotoxic hypoxia by increasing the physiological altitude. It has been observed that 1 ounce of alcohol can equate to about an additional 2,000 feet of physiological altitude, thus interfering with O_2 uptake and metabolism at the cellular level. Furthermore, the usual depressant effects of alcohol on behavior may cloud your recognition of your own degree of hypoxia, adding to your decreasing tolerance.

Fatigue

When you are mentally or physically fatigued you tolerate hypoxia poorly because you are already bordering on performance decrement. And because fatigue is a symptom of hypoxia, it becomes difficult to discriminate your level of hypoxia. You often erroneously reason that your fatigue is not a result of hypoxia and consequently do not take preventative actions, i.e., going on O_2.

Smoking

The CO in cigarette smoke is a serious threat to the pilot or flight attendant in flight. Carbon monoxide has an affinity for Hgb that is over 200 times more than that for O_2 and this results in hypemic hypoxia (Fig. 2-2). It has been noted by some that smoking three cigarettes in rapid succession, or smoking 20 to 30 cigarettes in a 24-hour period prior to flight may saturate from 8 to 10 percent of the Hgb in the body. In addition, approximately 20 percent of a smoker's night vision is lost, even at sea level. This can translate into a physiological altitude of an additional 3,000 to 5,000 feet.

Physical Fitness

If you are in good physical shape—that is, not overweight, have been exercising, and have a fairly nutritious diet—you are

Fig. 2-2 Smoking increases a pilot's physiological altitude.

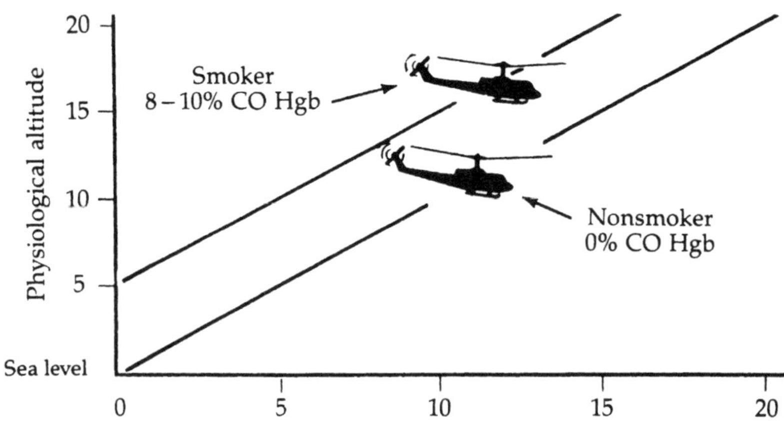

much more tolerant to the effects of low O_2 levels. The symptoms and potential incapacitation from hypoxia are still present, but you find them less severe, and more importantly, you are able to take appropriate action to recognize and avoid increasing hypoxia before you are truly at risk. In effect, the physiological ceiling is reduced. Also, keep in mind that it may be more than just improved tolerance. A healthy body is probably more efficient at using O_2 and therefore requires less O_2 for metabolic processes. Regardless, being in good physical condition is a true investment in maintaining a safe performance in flight. Being in less-than-optimal shape becomes a self-induced deterrent to tolerance.

Other Factors Affecting Response to Hypoxia

Several factors can determine the degree of hypoxia you can expect given the right circumstances. You have some control over these factors, but to a lesser degree, because they are a part of your flying environment and working conditions. When tolerance is described, it refers to how susceptible your body is to low levels of O_2. As a result of the following factors, you could become hypoxic at lower altitudes than you would expect, even if your controllable risk factors are absent.

Acclimatization

People who live at high altitudes develop an increased tolerance to the same conditions that would lead to hypoxia in people living at lower altitudes. Therefore, pilots and flight attendants who live in Denver (the "Mile High City") are more adapted to flying at a cabin altitude of 8,000 feet, or higher, than someone who lives in Los Angeles. Likewise, the LA-based crew who lands in Denver and has a layover there will already be slightly hypoxic when taking off the next day.

Absolute Altitude

The higher the altitude in the cabin (whether pressurized or not), the higher the risk of becoming hypoxic. Be advised that airline cabin altitude often reaches 8,000 feet. When the absolute altitude reaches a dangerous level, you must consider either lowering the cabin altitude or donning an O_2 mask.

Rate of Ascent

The quicker your cabin altitude climbs, the less effective your individual tolerance. Often, as a result of rapid ascent, you are even less aware of approaching hypoxia. The lack of time to notice suspicious symptoms often leads to an unexpected series of potentially incapacitating symptoms. In contrast, a slow ascent of cabin altitude, as with a slow leak, can be an insidious impairment without distinct symptoms.

Duration of Exposure

Staying at 8,000 feet for several hours (without supplemental O_2) could result in the same symptoms of compromised skills as ½ hour at about 16,000 feet. Symptoms are time related but also very unpredictable. As I will discuss later, the higher the altitude the shorter the exposure time needed before symptoms of hypoxia occur.

Ambient Temperature

Temperature extremes in the cockpit, especially in smaller recreational aircraft and poorly air-conditioned pressurized cabins, make your body less tolerant to diminished O_2 levels. Shivering when you are cold uses body energy and this increased activity requires more O_2. Coping with high heat and humidity also affects your tolerance because your body's circulatory system is working harder to maintain its core temperature.

Activity

Pilots are sedentary in the cockpit and physical exertion is often minimal. Flying without the help of an autopilot in turbulence can be exerting. Flight attendants, however, are physically more active than pilots and can expect some symptoms of hypoxia directly related to exertion. This is not a medical concern but it can be uncomfortable and distracting.

Time of Useful Consciousness (TUC)

The Time of Useful Conciousness (TUC) (also called effective performance time [EPT]) is the period of time you have from when O_2 becomes less available until you lose your ability to take action (e.g., getting on O_2 or going to a lower altitude) (Fig. 2-3). As described previously, a major symptom of hypoxia is euphoria and indifference. Therefore, if you go beyond your TUC, then you aren't even aware that you are in trouble and you will not take corrective action. The key words are *useful* and *effective*. You may be conscious but not making useful decisions.

The TUC decreases with increasing altitude and is dependent on the same tolerance factors defined previously. The TUC can be very short but only at cabin altitudes not frequently experienced. Decompression (sudden or slow loss of cabin pressure), however, still occurs in flight and you can quickly find yourself at altitudes in excess of 15,000 feet and not realize you have a shorter TUC. In fact, in a more rapid de-

Fig. 2-3 Time of useful consciousness decreases as the altitude increases.

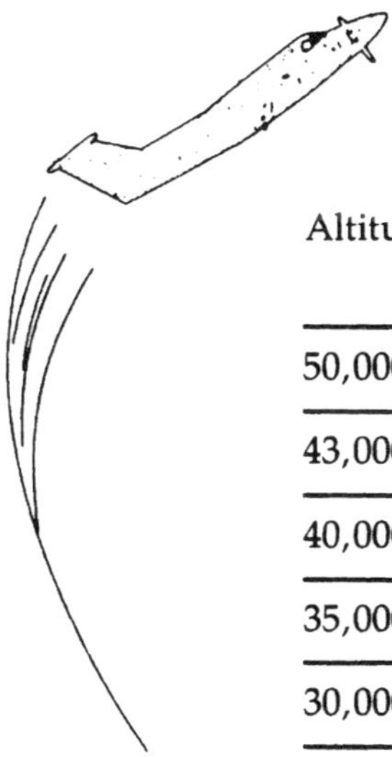

Altitude	Effective performance time	
50,000 feet and above	9 – 12	seconds
43,000	9 – 12	"
40,000	15 – 20	"
35,000	30 – 60	"
30,000	1 – 2	minutes
28,000	$2^1/_2$ – 3	"
25,000	4 – 6	"
22,000	8 – 10	"
18,000	20 – 30	"

compression, your TUC is shortened by one-third to one-half. Of greater concern, and more likely to occur, is subtle decompression, in which you are not aware that your cabin altitude is rising, resulting in a shortening TUC. For example, if you are flying without supplemental O_2 in a cabin where the altitude is slowly climbing to about 18,000 feet, you can easily get into trouble and not be aware of it. At this altitude the TUC is about 25 minutes. If you are busy and you are not keeping track of the time you are at this high altitude, you can quickly approach your TUC.

Prevention of Hypoxia

There is nothing remarkable about preventing hypoxia. As already discussed, avoidance of conditions that increase the risk of becoming hypoxic is paramount. Hypoxia also is prevented by maintaining a high level of suspicion anytime your cabin altitude is above 5,000 feet, especially at night. Like maintenance of the aircraft, preventive physiological management is more productive than crisis management. Waiting for symptoms of hypoxia to be observed before you take action is crisis management. Prevention of hypoxia, therefore, becomes anticipation of becoming hypoxic under conditions where hypoxia can happen. If you are a smoker, moderate drinker, and physically out of shape, you are at greater risk even at lower altitudes.

The obvious solution is to be in a pressurized cabin at an altitude of less than 10,000 feet or to use an O_2 mask. According to regulations, you might be legal without O_2 at 10,000 feet but you also can be subtly incapacitated. Many commercial pilots who experience cabin altitudes of 7,000 feet or more go on O_2 just before they begin a descent, especially after a long flight at night.

Treatment of Hypoxia

If there is any suspicion of hypoxia in yourself or a crewmate, the immediate use of 100 percent O_2 is essential. Aside from the rare occurrence of O_2 toxicity, you cannot hurt anyone by giving him or her O_2. If someone is hypoxic, then response and recovery will be almost immediate. If there isn't an immediate improvement, you must think of other causes for the symptoms. If supplemental O_2 is not available, get the airplane or cabin altitude below 10,000 feet. This is a valid reason to declare an emergency to ATC.

Hyperventilation

Hyperventilation is simply breathing too rapidly, which results in exhaling dangerous amounts of CO_2 during respiration. The symptoms are seldom incapacitating but hyperventilation does produce, at the very least, a potentially serious distraction, often in a busy cockpit. Therefore, the problem is only further aggravated by increasing anxiety level and breathing rate. It becomes a vicious circle.

Causes

Fear, stress, and anxiety can cause you to override normal automatic functions of respiration, such as breathing rate. As you become more stressed, you tend to breathe faster. Because you are more apt to observe this in others than in yourself, this is another reason for depending on and trusting your crewmates.

Symptoms

Unfortunately, many of the symptoms of hyperventilation are similar to those experienced in hypoxia, fainting, and decompression sickness. They include, but are not limited to, tingling sensations in your fingers, toes, and around the lips; small muscle spasms; hot and cold sensations; visual impairment; dizziness, and, in severe cases, unconsciousness. The challenge is to make the proper diagnosis based on the symptoms and then take appropriate action.

If hyperventilation is suspected, trying to get voluntary control of your breathing rate is the most effective method of treatment. Normal breathing rate is about 12 to 16 breaths per minute. Recognizing that excess CO_2 is exhaled by rapid breathing, using the paper bag method also helps. Breathing into the bag makes you concentrate on slowing your breathing rate as well as rebreathing CO_2. Because hypoxia and hyperventilation have similar symptoms and hypoxia can cause you to hyperventilate, the initial treatment for these symptoms is the same—O_2. A good rule of thumb, therefore, is to go on 100 percent O_2, and get your mind off your anxiety by working on something or mentally figuring out a problem. Even singing or talking has been suggested.

Final Thoughts on Hypoxia

It is essential that there be a mutual understanding and respect by all aircrew for hypoxia and hyperventilation. You should expect your crewmate to watch you just as you are obligated to keep your suspicions up in hypoxia-generating conditions. This is true for all facets of aviation, including helicopter flight, where there is a false sense of security as a result of the perception that you aren't going to get high enough to become hypoxic. Helicopters are flying higher all the time, in excess of 30,000 feet! This is a common occurrence in mountainous areas where you can leave sea level and quickly be at an altitude in excess of 15,000 feet. Although flying less than 10,000 feet AGL is common, remember that your physiological altitude can be much higher, especially if you are at the higher altitude

Hypoxia Prayer

Be with us now, O Lord. And when
We're told to breathe thy oxygen
From dangling masks, be with us then.

Be near us, Lord. We know that flight
Is but a challenge to thy might,
A privilege and not a right.

O Lord, whose mercy we revere,
We know we shouldn't be up here.

(*The Punch Book of Travel*, 1974)

for extended periods. Hypoxia happens, even to professionals. It needn't be a dramatic or obvious event. Subtle performance impairment takes place even with minimal hypoxia.

Poisons in the Air

Carbon Monoxide

Carbon monoxide is colorless, odorless, tasteless, and slightly lighter than air. The effects of CO are subtle and deadly. Carbon monoxide poisoning is more common than poisoning by any other toxic gas. Like in hypoxia, CO poisoning is painless and can incapacitate you before you know you are in trouble. Carbon monoxide is present in every smoker's body.

Effects of Exposure
Relatively low concentrations of CO in the air can, in time, produce very high blood concentrations. It is a cumulative problem. Such accumulations can occur in less than 30 minutes at CO levels in the air of only 0.5 percent. Carbon monoxide competes with O_2 for attachment to Hgb, which leads to hypemic hypoxia, even at low altitudes.

Symptoms
Like in hypoxia, the symptoms of CO intoxication are often subjective. They include headache, weakness, nervousness, tremors, and ultimately unconsciousness. As expected, a loss of visual acuity also occurs, especially with night and peripheral vision.

Treatment
The treatment for CO poisoning is immediate 100 percent O_2. Unlike with hypoxia, this treatment is an extremely slow process. It can take several days for high CO concentrations in the blood to be reduced to normal levels. Although the symptoms of hypoxic hypoxia and CO poisoning are alike, going on 100 percent O_2 will not immediately relieve CO poisoning symptoms. This is another clue to determine why you or your crewmate feels impaired. Medical attention should be sought if there is any doubt about the reasons for the symptoms.

Cabin Decompression

Decompression occurs when cabin pressure is lost for any reason, suddenly or slowly. The cabin altitude decompresses to the ambient pressure within which your airplane is flying. Thus, if the cabin is pressurized to 6,000 feet and you are flying at 20,000 feet and a leak develops, your cabin can suddenly (or slowly) be at 20,000 feet. Recall that your TUC also will become shorter as the decompression continues.

One characteristic of a rapid decompression is a loud popping or dull banging sound. Concurrently, there is usually flying debris, paper, and dust mostly, with some items being sucked out of the aircraft as the air under pressure in the airplane rushes out the hole into lower pressure. Fogging is very common and sometimes confused with smoke. The temperature suddenly drops to equalize the outside temperature. This temperature change can obviously be incapacitating because ambient temperature at 35,000 feet is about –67°F. The combination of cold and hypoxia can quickly become an emergency.

Subtle decompression could be considered the most potentially dangerous type of decompression because you may not be aware that your cabin altitude is increasing. Not all pressurized airplanes give warning about cabin ascent rate or indicate that a dangerous cabin altitude has been reached. Decompressions can occur even in modern aircraft.

The most noticeable effect of all but the subtle decompressions is the sudden rush of air from the lungs. There may be trapped gas problems, but they should not be significant unless it's an explosive decompression. Having a cold or flu increases the risk of problems. The primary concern is the sudden exposure to extreme hypoxic and cold conditions, especially at high altitudes. The treatment remains the same: Get on O_2 and get to a lower altitude and, of course, fly the airplane.

Ear Blocks and Other Problems

Your body can withstand tremendous changes in pressure as long as the air pressure in your body cavities is able to equalize with that of the ambient air. Thus, the pressure inside any cavity or organ of your body where gas is present does not cause any problems unless the pressure is not the same as the pressure surrounding that cavity or organ. Problems occur when the expanding (or contracting) gas within your body cannot escape to allow ambient and body pressures to equalize. When gases within body fluids, such as blood, escape from the fluid and enter your body (evolved gas), this causes the bends.

Dysbarism is a synonym often used for the bends and sometimes associated with trapped gas. It is no longer an accepted term because it is nonspecific. It is better to use the terms *trapped gas*, *ear* or *sinus blocks*, and *evolved gas disorders*.

As a result of a greater differential in pressure per thousand feet at lower altitudes, the risk of developing any kind of block is higher below 15,000 feet. Thus, a rapid descent from 30,000 feet to 20,000 feet often causes little or no discomfort, whereas a similar rate of descent from 15,000 feet to 5,000 feet causes considerable distress. The greatest pressure change (differential) is from sea level to 5,000 feet and this is where most blocks occur. Ear and sinus blocks also are noticed in self-contained underwater breathing apparatus (scuba) diving where the most significant pressure changes occur in the first 15 to 30 feet of water.

Middle Ear Block (Barotitis)

During ascent and as the ambient air pressure is reduced, the expanding air within the middle ear is intermittently released through the eustachian tube (Fig. 2-4). During descent the same process should take place, but air movement is in the opposite direction. This equalization of pressure on either side of the eardrum is essential for proper hearing because the flexibility of your eardrum must not be compromised. As the pressure increases in the middle ear, a small bubble forms that, after it reaches a certain size, escapes through your eustachian tube. You can often feel this equalization of pressure as the air bubble pops.

This pressure equalization should be automatic without any conscious effort, especially under ideal conditions. Normal swallowing often clears the ears. Problems arise when your eu-

Fig. 2-4 Common methods of clearing an ear block won't work if the block is the result of the mucous membranes being swollen from a cold or hayfever.

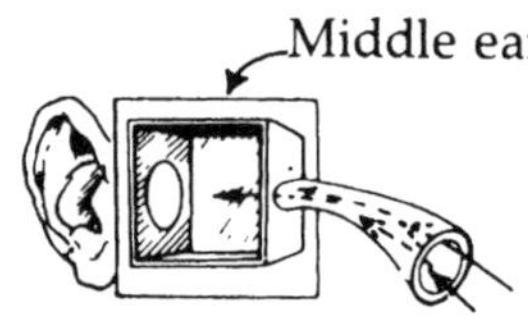

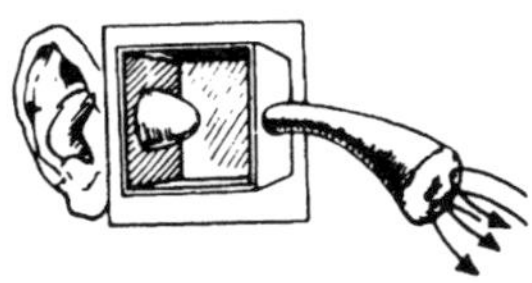

stachian tube does not allow passage of air, usually a result of the mucous membranes inside the eustachian tube being swollen from a cold or hayfever. Often, the passage of air is only outward and not back into the middle ear—like a one-way valve.

An unexpected, delayed cause of a block occurs when breathing O_2, as in unpressurized cabins at altitudes requiring O_2-breathing masks. Here, pure, undiluted O_2 enters the cavity. If a block occurs and it is unable to be cleared, the cavity is pressurized with O_2 that, in turn, is absorbed by the mucous membranes. Now, instead of high pressure, a lower pressure develops with equally disabling symptoms. This phenomenon is fairly frequent in passengers who sleep through the flight (their swallowing rate decreases during sleep) or who are not actively clearing their ears. During descent they develop a mild block. Ear blocks also occur in nonpressurized aircraft where you are breathing O_2 on a long cross-country. In all these situations, however, the real problem occurs a few hours later, when you are on the ground because the O_2 has been absorbed in the still-blocked ear. The pain returns and it may even be worse. Now it's time to see the doctor.

Symptoms

Inability to clear your ears (equalize pressure) can result in conditions ranging from mild discomfort to severe pain in the middle ear, often radiating to the side of your head. A true disabling earache. Ask anyone who has ever had an ear block and you will know someone who never wants to experience it again. It is worse than a severe toothache. The pain becomes worse as the pressure changes and it does not always go away even after you have landed. Sometimes, the trapped gas within the middle ear reaches a pressure high enough that the eardrum ruptures. The good news is that the pain then instantly goes away but you will have a tear in your eardrum and need treatment by a physician.

Ear blocks primarily occur on descent and often clear themselves on ascent because the nasal end of the eustachian tube acts like a one-way valve for air passage. The Valsalva maneuver helps keep this valve open, if performed soon enough.

Whatever the cause of the ear block, you are disabled and potentially incapacitated by it. At the very least, you are distracted from flying duties. Your ears can be physically damaged, sometimes permanently. Despite continuing awareness of the causes of ear blocks and their associated dangers, pilots and aircrew still get into trouble with them. A major cause is flying with a cold and delaying the use of techniques to clear your ears. Scuba divers know to begin clearing their ears at the first indication of a block. Aviators must do the same.

Treatment and Prevention

The best treatment for a medical problem is to prevent it from happening. I've indicated that flying with a cold or congestion is like asking for trouble, yet many pilots fly under these conditions. Admittedly, only a few develop a serious block but that infrequent event is a major risk to safe flight.

In reality, if every pilot grounded himself or herself for every sniffle, there would be few pilots available to fly. Therefore, if you have mild congestion (and there is no good definition of *mild*) then taking some decongestant medication before you begin the flight might be appropriate. This treatment must not contain antihistamines! Some long-acting cortisone-type nose sprays also might allow you to fly safely. The dilemma is that, technically, no medications are legal or safe if they could cause side effects that might compromise your performance or incapacitate you in any way. Most aviation medical examiners (AMEs) should be able to help you decide, but the ultimate decision and responsibility is yours.

If you are prone to early ear blocks, it might be wise to carry a small bottle of a long-acting decongestant nose spray in your flight bag. This spray should be used only when you sense a block developing inflight but still early enough that the spray has a chance to take effect. All other measures should still be used to relieve the block.

Traditional and safe methods of clearing the block are without medication. The most common is to move the jaw and swallow at the same time. Chewing gum is a great way to accomplish this movement. Yawning, moving your head around, or a combination often clears the ears.

Another technique and probably the most effective, is the Valsalva maneuver. As soon as a block begins to develop (i.e., you sense some mild pressure in your ears), hold the fleshy part of your nose tight (as if you were going to jump into a pool of water). Then blow hard against your nose (as if you wanted to blow your nose). These actions often lead to an increase in the pressure within the nasal area and force air back into the middle ear through the eustachian tube. It is not likely (but it is possible if you over do it) that you can blow hard enough to injure your eardrums, so blow fairly hard. This procedure is the same one that is used by scuba divers when descending into water.

If all these attempts fail, consider taking the aircraft (or cabin altitude) higher, to a level above where the block began. Then begin a very slow descent, using the techniques already mentioned, but now under controlled conditions, keeping ahead of the pressure change.

If a block persists after landing, see your doctor. Unresolved blocks can lead to inflammation and sometimes an infection. A middle ear infection will temporarily ground you.

Sinus Block (Barosinusitis)

Just like in your ears, air blocks also can occur in your sinuses, except the openings to the sinus cavities are much smaller and the Valsalva technique is not as effective. The pain from a sinus block is as incapacitating as that of an ear block, and often more so. A sinus block feels like "an ice pick in the face." All the more reason to be cautious about flying with a cold or hayfever. Additionally, unlike the middle ear, the sinuses are affected by both ascent and descent.

Teeth (Barodontalgia)

Common sources of barodontalgia are cavities, abscesses, and inadequate fillings. Pain often increases with altitude and may become disabling. Descent usually brings some relief. Dental intervention is essential once you recognize that you had such a block. Explain to the dentist what the circumstances are relating to the tooth pain. If it feels as if the entire top row of teeth is hurting, or if the discomfort occurs on descent, it is probably a sinus block (maxillary sinus) rather than barodontalgia.

The Bends

Evolved gas disorders, the physiological or physical events that occur with variations in pressure, are known by different names. Such disorders are often minimized by the aviation community because it is thought that they only occur in military fighter pilots and divers. Scuba divers are very aware of what can happen to the gases dissolved in the blood when they are released under lower ambient pressures. Evolved gas disorders, however, can and do occur in flight crew, although more slowly and at much higher altitudes. The following is some of the terminology used when discussing evolved gas disorders.

Decompression Sickness (DCS)

Decompression sickness is the generic medical term used to identify all degrees and variations of evolved gas disorders, excluding trapped gas disorders. Decompression sickness includes conditions that result when gases dissolved within the blood and tissues are released as the surrounding pressure decreases. This release of gas results in small bubbles being transported by the blood to various organs and other parts of your body.

Aeroembolism

An aeroembolism involves air (as a bubble) that is acting as an embolism or blockage that can move throughout your body. An embolism often means a blood clot but generally can include anything that could obstruct a blood vessel, such as a bubble of air.

Bends

The bends is the most common term used in discussing DCS, especially in scuba. It is one kind of DCS, specifically involving the joints. It does not, however, refer to the other kinds of DCS, which are actually more dangerous. Decompression sickness usually refers to involvement of the nervous system. In actuality, the bends is by far the most common type (over 85%) of DCS.

Basic Physiology

Henry's Gas Law states that the amount of gas dissolved in a solution is directly proportional to the pressure of that gas over the solution. This law can be demonstrated by observing what happens when you remove the top or pull the tab on a bottle or can of soda pop or beer. As you know, the contents are under pressure. When that pressure is released, so is the gas (in this example, CO_2) and bubbles immediately form and come to the surface. Nitrogen dissolved in the blood responds the same way. As the pressure outside the body decreases, gas is evolved from the blood and is transported as bubbles throughout the body.

Interestingly, fat tissue dissolves five to six times more N_2 than blood. Thus, the extra fat that some pilots have covering their body and internal organs is an additional source of N_2

that puts him or her at increased risk of developing DCS at higher altitudes. The same is true for flight passengers.

Physiologically, these gases, especially N_2, have the potential of being released into the bloodstream as pressures change over time. For example, inhaled air at sea level is absorbed into tissues and blood. After ascending to higher cabin altitudes (greater than 18,000 feet) and staying there for a few hours, some of these gases are released into the blood. Gas bubbles are formed until the cabin altitude returns to sea level. The symptoms that result from these bubbles blocking blood flow, along with the effects on your body, are what concern you when you fly at these altitudes.

Effects on the Body

Circulatory System

Gas bubbles can act as a blockage within smaller vessels and are called *embolisms*. Such blockage is of minimal consequence until the bubble gets larger or more vessels become blocked. The ultimate problem exists in your body's organs.

Musculoskeletal System

Gas bubbles can cause pain in your larger joints, such as in the knee, shoulders, and elbows. The pain is often described as a gnawing ache, ranging from mild to severe, and obviously either distracting or incapacitating in the cockpit. This condition is also called the bends. The pain tends to be progressive, especially as ascent is continued. There is also the tendency for pain to recur in the same location during subsequent flights. It may involve several joints at the same time. Achy joints are common in everyone and there has to be a high index of suspicion that the discomfort could be DCS and not arthritis or a sprain.

Paresthesias

Paresthesias involves the nerves, causing abnormal sensations such as tingling, itching, and cold and warm feelings. It is thought that these reactions are from the bubbles forming locally around nerve tracts in the skin. Such symptoms also are common in hypoxia and hyperventilation, which means you must be aware of your environment. You must consider which condition has the greatest chance of occurring before deciding a course of action. Another term is *skin manifestations of DCS.*

Chokes

The symptoms of the chokes occur in the chest (thorax) and lungs. Gas bubbles intrude on the pulmonary vessels (blood vessels carrying blood into the lung tissue). The first signs are a burning sensation mid chest (sternum) that progresses to a stabbing pain accentuated by deep breathing. It is similar to the feeling after a sudden burst of exercise when it is difficult to catch your breath. There is an almost uncontrollable need to cough, but coughing is ineffective at relieving the pain and doesn't produce any sputum. Finally, there is a feeling of suffocation, with typical signs of cyanosis (decreased O_2 supply). Immediate descent is necessary because a potential medical emergency exists. If no intervention takes place, you may collapse into unconsciousness. After getting to the ground, you will often still be fatigued and have a sore chest for several hours.

Disorders of the Brain (CNS)

Although uncommon, brain disorders are very serious. When the brain and spinal cord are exposed to N_2 bubbles, the most common symptoms are visual, such as flashing or flickering lights. Headaches, paralysis, inability to hear or speak, and disorientation also occur. Any of these symptoms (in the appropriate conditions of flight) should be highly suspect and are considered a medical emergency. Brain disorder symptoms are easily confused with those of hypoxia and pulling Gs. Keeping a high index of suspicion is important if you are flying at altitude for an extended period of time.

Prevention

Decompression sickness is relatively uncommon in typical flying. The bends do occur, however, in unpressurized, smaller aircraft flying at altitudes above 15,000 feet, even though O_2 is being used. Therefore, if you are in conditions of high cabin altitudes or know you will reach such altitudes (even in a helicopter going from sea level to mountaintop rescues), anticipate that you could be affected.

Factors Affecting Severity

If you think you are susceptible to DCS, awareness of the following factors should help prevent serious problems.

Time at Altitude

The longer you are at excessive altitude, the greater the risk for developing DCS. More gas bubbles can form and be transported throughout your body under such altitudes.

Rate of Ascent

The more rapid the ascent, the greater the chance of bubble formation because your body has little time to equalize the pressure changes.

Altitude

The threshold for developing DCS is usually above 18,000 feet. It increases more rapidly above 26,000 feet.

Age and Obesity

Older people tend to be more susceptible to DCS than younger people, even under low-risk conditions. The same is true for obese people whose fat can store more gas, especially N_2. It is also suspected that recent alcohol use can increase the risk of DCS.

Exercise and Injury

Exercise is one of the most important factors influencing susceptibility to DCS, whereas injury is of lesser importance. It is wise not to exert yourself prior to a flight or immediately after one at high altitude.

Repeated Exposure

Several flights over a short period of time (48 hours) increase the chances of DCS problems. Repeated insults to affected organs make them more susceptible.

In the civilian world (military is the exception), the chances of developing DCS are small. If you are caught at altitude in IFR in a nonpressurized airplane, and make several trips within a 2-day period, however, you could be a prime candidate for DCS. Keep this in mind, especially if you are a scuba diver.

Scuba Diving

Decompression sickness is a familiar term to scuba divers. Divers are more susceptible to DCS than aircrew because there is a greater differential in pressure in water and in shorter distances. For example, the pressure in water doubles at 30 feet, whereas in flight you have to go from 18,000 feet to sea level to double the pressure.

What happens is that at only 33 feet in water, your body absorbs twice as much N_2 from the scuba air tank (the tank does not carry O_2, only pressurized air). Every diver knows this and anticipates problems when returning to the surface. Prevention involves understanding the diving table, known to all divers, which determines the steps to take to prevent DCS. These steps do not include climbing into an airplane and essentially further decreasing the pressure surrounding the body.

Therefore, a rule of thumb: Don't take one more dive before leaving for home in a plane whose cabin altitude is probably around 8,000 feet. The same situation is present as if you were flying at 40,000 feet unpressurized! The recommended waiting time is 12 hours after the last dive and at least 24 hours if you were a part of a dive that required a controlled ascent (decompression stop dive). Current studies are suggesting that these times should be increased.

If DCS is suspected in a scuba diver, then that diver must get to a hyperbaric chamber (recompression) and be monitored by medical personnel. The dive shop should have the number of your closest chamber for treatment through an organization called Divers Alert Network (DAN).

Altitude Chamber Ride

An altitude chamber ride is a common experience for military aircrew and is offered to the civilian pilot, although not required by the FAA. It is highly recommended that you have at least one chamber ride for the following reasons.

1. You experience basic symptoms of hypoxia and decompression.
2. You recognize personal symptoms before they become disabling. Because everyone responds differently to the same conditions, it is important to recognize your unique symptoms. Only through the chamber ride can you determine your signs and symptoms.
3. Experience rapid decompression (R/D) in controlled conditions and realize that it is not the terrifying situation you might have imagined. Also, it helps you realize the shock of a R/D and how it can immobilize you and hinder your reactions.
4. Gain confidence in and respect for high-altitude flight, especially for the insidious affects of hypoxia.

The ride profile may vary but basically you are taken to altitude, experience hypoxia and trapped gas, are shown the effects on other participants so that you can detect these problems in others, and then are brought down (Fig. 2-5). The most useful part of the chamber ride is to be able to recognize your own symptoms of early stage hypoxia so that you can take immediate action (get on O_2) before you are unaware that you are disabled or incapacitated. You also are shown what it is like to pressure breathe and the effect of hypoxia on night vision. The FAA's chamber ride is free. Give them a call or check with your AME.

Fig. 2-5 Every pilot should take at least one altitude chamber flight in his or her career.

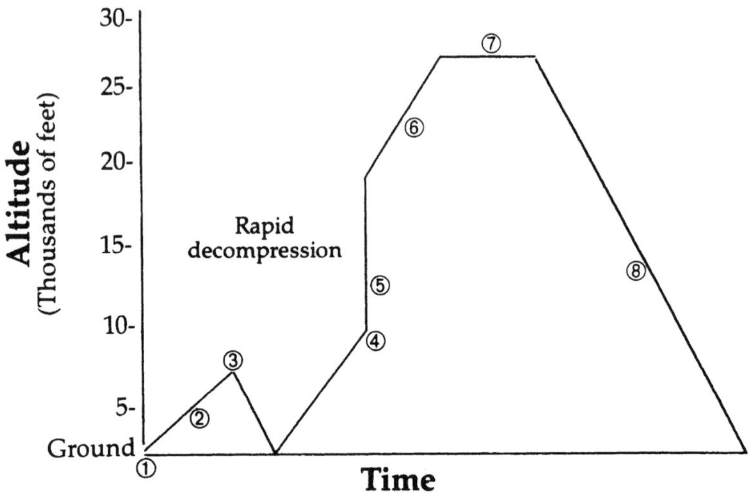

Altitude chamber flight profile

1. Preflight briefing.
2. Mask fitting and operation of oxygen regulator and intercom system in chamber.
3. Ascend to 6,000 feet and descend to ground level to determine proper clearing of ears and sinus cavities. Rate of ascent and descent is 3,000 feet per minute.
4. Re-ascend to 8,000 feet at a rate of 3,000 feet per minute.
5. Rapid decompression (8 – 10 seconds) from 8,000 feet to 18,000 feet. Masks will be donned during the decompression.
6. Ascend to 25,000 feet at the rate of 3,500 feet per minute.
7. Removal of masks at 25,000 feet to enable trainees to experience symptoms of hypoxia. Five minutes time limit off supplemental oxygen.
8. Descend to ground level at the rate of 3,000 feet per minute. Trainees will practice pressure breathing and discuss their hypoxia symptoms on descent.

Disorientation in Flight 3

There were numerous towering cumulous clouds, none of them threatening, but they were impossible to avoid. John, who was at the controls, was tired from a party last night and was mentally absorbed with his young son's recent surgery. He was IFR rated but had not flown in real instrument conditions for several months. On a few occasions, while inadvertently entering a cloud, he noticed he came out in the clear in less than a wings-level attitude. But he was more concerned about getting home than how well he was flying. The next cloud he entered got his attention because it was bigger than anticipated. He looked at his instruments and realized he was in a climbing turn but it felt like he was descending. He began to correct the aircraft's attitude but realized too late that it was getting worse. He entered clear air in an uncontrollable spin.

AS PREVIOUSLY STATED, the greatest challenge to you and your fitness to fly is the prevention of a medical incapacitation. If you, your passengers, and the FAA could be guaranteed that you or your crew would not become incapacitated in flight—providing the airplane works—the aviation community would have few concerns about safety. There is, however, an exception and that is becoming disoriented.

If your plane works, and you are not impaired medically, then the only other significant performance factor in getting safely from point A to point B is maintaining orientation of the plane and yourself relative to the horizon and placement in space. Orientation (and awareness of your situation) is the key element in accident and incident prevention. Situation awareness (SA), a term used in conjunction with orientation, involves an awareness of what's going on around you with other aircraft, your location, weather, ATC, etc. Lack of orientation is called *disorientation*, and disorientation, in various forms, can be a common occurrence on any flight. Disorientation can be temporal, postural, vestibular, positional, auditory, or spatial, all of which, by themselves or in combination, can make an otherwise uneventful flight a memorable experience.

Disorientation is a human factor, not helped much by the advanced technology of electronic guidance systems and glass cockpits. Disorientation is a leading cause (not just a contributing factor) for more than 15 percent of aviation accidents and incidents. All pilots experience disorientation at one time or another and most situations go unreported, both in military and civilian aviation. In most cases, the pilot and crew recover from the disorientation and no one is the wiser.

Because few such scenarios are officially reported, disorientation does not show up in human factors statistics as frequently as it actually occurs. But if you listen to your colleagues talk in the crew lounge, you will recognize that disorientation is occurring frequently. Because you know disorientation occurs, it is your responsibility to take measures to prevent disorientation by maintaining an awareness of what affects orientation in the flight environment and by keeping current in flight proficiency. Experiencing the effects of disorientation through unusual attitude flight or Vertigon simulators reinforces the power of this human factor.

Therefore, the objective of this chapter is to raise your level of awareness, to identify conditions that lead to the various kinds of disorientation, and to discuss measures to minimize the occurrence of disorientation in your flying experiences. Intolerance to confusing signals from the body is increased even if you are only minimally impaired physiologically, thus increasing your risk of becoming disorientated. You can easily become disoriented for a variety of reasons. Like a graveyard spiral, these cumulative factors eventually lead to a performance problem sufficient enough to cause an accident or incident.

Types of Disorientation

To be oriented in any and all situations requires that you are mentally aware of your physical reference to a particular point. It follows that if you aren't oriented to a particular point, then you may experience disorientation. This is just plain common sense. There are several senses the body uses to orient itself. Vision is the most important, followed by vestibular (inner ear), and proprioceptive (relative muscle position) inputs, respectively. The placement of sound also helps maintain orientation. I will discuss each input in terms of how it can give proper, accurate, yet occasionally misleading cues, often working in harmony. Many times, however, there is a conflict, or disharmony, between these cues, from their different sources, and your perception of how well you are doing, thus creating more confusion.

Postural Disorientation

A constant source of sensory input comes from your body's interpretation of the direction of gravitational force through proprioceptive signals—positional signals from various muscles and tendons in your body. Your mind is programmed to interpret these signals as being up or down, relative to the earth and its gravitational pull. This input, in turn, determines your posture, or your position relative to the ground. Concurrently, there are proprioceptive sensors within your skin, muscles, tendons, and joints that detect changes in relative position, pressure, and changes from that of up or down.

Indications of Loss of Situation Awareness

- No one looking out windows.
- No one flying.
- When expectations of events are not met.
- Pilot or crew unsure of condition of aircraft.
- Two or more sources of independent information don't agree.
- When confusion, questions, or statements of concern are not resolved.
- Attention of crew focused on one item, event, or condition to exclusion of all other activity.
- When consideration is given to using an undocumented procedure.
- When consideration is given to violating minimums.

Proprioceptive signals are generated every time a muscle contracts or relaxes, tendons are pulled or released, and joints move. All these inputs, continuously coming to your brain, tell you your position, usually relative to the common foundation of gravity. It's similar to INS navigation whereby avionics determines your plane's current position relative to where it started the flight.

Another source of signals defining posture is part of your vestibular system and your otolith organs, located in your inner ear. When your body is subjected to up and down changes, these signals play a role, along with proprioception, in determining your position. This group of signals is discussed under vestibular orientation.

Because you perceive gravity as "down," any input from proprioception or the otolith organs is interpreted as either being down or a variation from that position. Your largest source of such information is realized when you are sitting down; hence "seat of the pants" flying. Comfortable postural orientation in flight is felt in a well-coordinated turn, during which all postural signals are indicating that you are sitting upright, directly related to gravity. If your turn is coordinated and doesn't disrupt your vestibular system, and your position also is confirmed visually, there is no impairment to your perception of performance.

In an improperly executed turn, especially in a climb, these signals become very confusing to your brain, giving false illusions as to your true posture. Rather than being pushed into the seat, your body is pushed sideways as in a skid or slip, giving the impression of tilting. In the absence of visual reference, the only sensation you experience is your body being pressed into the seat, but not necessarily toward the ground. For example, recovering from such a situation in a climb gives the illusion of descending, causing you to pull back on the stick.

Positional Disorientation

Positional disorientation basically means that you are lost, if even for a brief moment, and you don't know your position. You become disoriented until you can resolve where you are and where you are heading. Thus, for a while, you don't know what to do. Do you keep going, go back, call for directions, or what? Positional disorientation also is called *geographic* or *directional disorientation*. No matter what the terminology, they all mean the same thing—you are temporarily lost!

All animals are creatures of habit, especially humans. Much of what you do, day after day, is a routine that you do the same way and usually without too much thought. Interrupt that routine and you are disoriented, not knowing how to continue without having to think about it. For example, consider how you take a shower (or bath). You wash yourself in the same way, each time starting at one part of your body and ending up at another. If you start with the front of your left shoulder, that's how you start every time.

To demostrate how you can become disoriented, when you next wash yourself, change the sequence. Start with your right foot. Now you have to think about what to wash next. This is no longer your routine and for a moment you are lost on your own body. You are briefly disoriented.

The same thing happens on familiar routes. You fly the same airways, talk to the same controllers, and make the same approaches on all the legs of the trip. Initially, when you fly the route for the first time, you concentrate on maintaining your awareness of where you are. Then the trip truly becomes routine—there is nothing to break the monotony of the hundredth trip. It now becomes easy to fall into the trap of passing a checkpoint, or flying right by it without knowing it. If ATC gives you a revised flight plan or changes your heading for traffic, you may miss the new clearance and continue on the same flight path you have always used. Or you may set up your approach to the wrong airport or runway. Pilots have been known to land at an airport not in their flight plan.

You become more susceptible to positional disorientation if you are distracted. You may be thinking about problems at home, concentrating on some activity in the cockpit unrelated to flying (reading a manual or listening to a commercial radio station), or having a conversation with a crewmate. Now both of you are out of the loop of maintaining positional awareness. And it's much worse if you are fatigued.

Another trap is the return flight or "get-homitis." This becomes more pervasive than the initial leg because there is the added distraction of anticipating what needs to be done at home. Your checklists that were read many times before become superficially reviewed. Distances, checkpoints, and waypoints become committed to memory (or so you think). Even familiar frequencies are part of this virtually automatic flight. Now throw in any deviation from the expected routine, or a malfunction of the aircraft, and you are easily disoriented. You have to spend time reasoning out what needs to be done to correct the problem and get back on course.

Pride often gets in the way when you think that you can get out of this fix without having to refer to manuals or maps. Certainly you may be reluctant to admit to ATC or even to a crewmate that you are lost or forgot the controlling center's frequency. Consider how this situation can be amplified if, at the same time, you enter actual instrument conditions. This combination of positional and potential vestibular disorientation is an incident or accident waiting to happen.

Temporal Disorientation

Disorientation relative to time (also called *temporal disorientation*) is subjective. We each perceive time differently under different situations. How long an activity lasts in your mind depends on the level of activity and interest occurring at that time. Time can be perceived as being expanded; that is, you think you have more time to accomplish some action. Likewise, time may appear to be compressed with you feeling that more time has passed than in actuality. This is common in monotonous, slow, and uninteresting activities.

It is not known in full how the mind perceives time. There is some evidence that the amount of adrenaline flowing through your body determines how much time is perceived as available in your mind.

Adrenaline (and cortisone) are chemicals that are released under fight-or-flight situations, allowing your body to respond quickly to unexpected and emergency situations. With extra emergency adrenaline, blood flow is shunted to critical organs such as muscles, heart, and brain, and pulse rate and blood pressure increase. Your brain now becomes more intensely alert and processes information at an accelerated rate in high activity.

Whatever the reason, the perception of time expansion is real in your mind during the critical event. It becomes a concern because in an emergency you may take too long to react, thinking that there is plenty of time available to try some other course of action.

The opposite is true in situations of decreased mental and physical activity. Time drags on although you feel it is moving faster. This perception is less critical than that of time expansion in flight because the actual prolonged time makes the trip even more boring. It doesn't greatly affect performance other than by increasing the likelihood of positional disorientation. Furthermore, this perception can add to an already boring trip, leading your mind to wander from the duties at hand.

Vestibular Disorientation

Spatial disorientation is commonly used to explain what is actually vestibular disorientation. Although they often occur at the same time and are a source of impairment, they are different and occur under different situations. *Vertigo* is also used to describe the symptoms, but in reality this term, to the medical profession, is related to a medical disorder that is a cause for medical certification denial until proven otherwise.

Now that I've confused you, let's explain the differences and why it is important to differentiate between the two for yourself as well as when you are discussing the topic of disorientation. Vestibular disorientation will be explained first and then spatial disorientation.

The vestibular system is located in the inner ear (Fig. 3-1). This system consists of two distinct structures, the otolith organs, which sense linear acceleration and gravity, and the semicircular canals, which sense angular acceleration.

Otolith Organs

Changes in the position of your head relative to the gravitational force cause the otolithic granules to shift within the fluid of the organ, giving the sensation of the pull of gravity as they move downward (Fig. 3-2). In a steady state, these granules don't move. If for any reason these granules are in motion, you perceive that there has been a change in your position relative to true gravity.

Fig. 3-1 Anatomy of the ear.

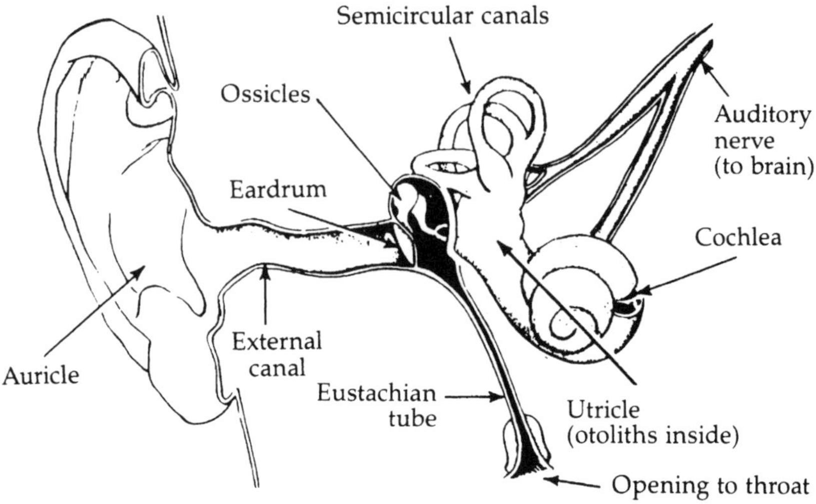

Fig. 3-2 Semicircular canal.

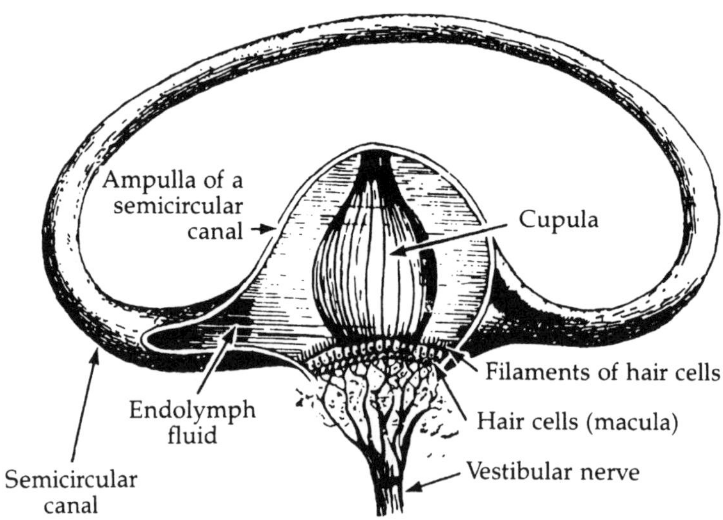

Semicircular Canals

This organ responds to roll, pitch, and yaw. It is similar in perception to three gyros in three planes of direction perpendicular to each other (Fig. 3-3). Bending of the cupula results in movement of the hair cells situated beneath the cupula. (These

Fig. 3-3 Hair cells change position during turns.

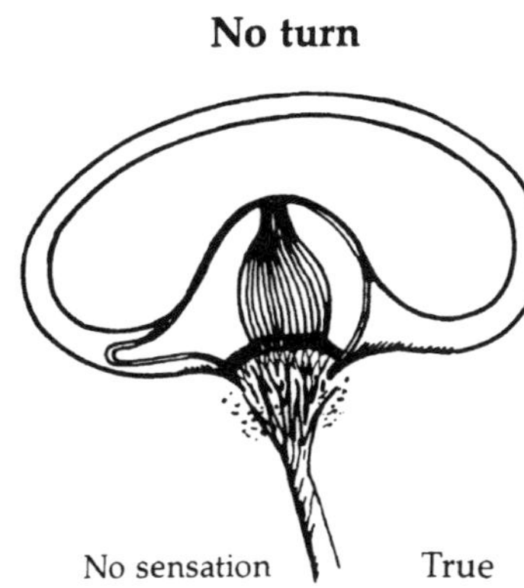

Hair cell position and resulting sensation under nonacceleration conditions.

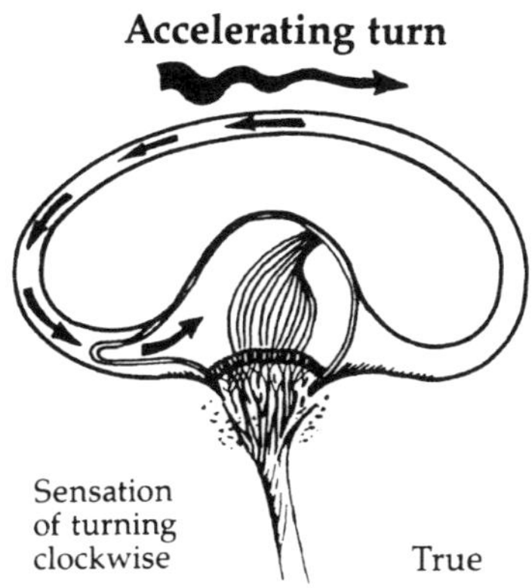

Hair cell position and resulting sensation under conditions of acceleration to the right.

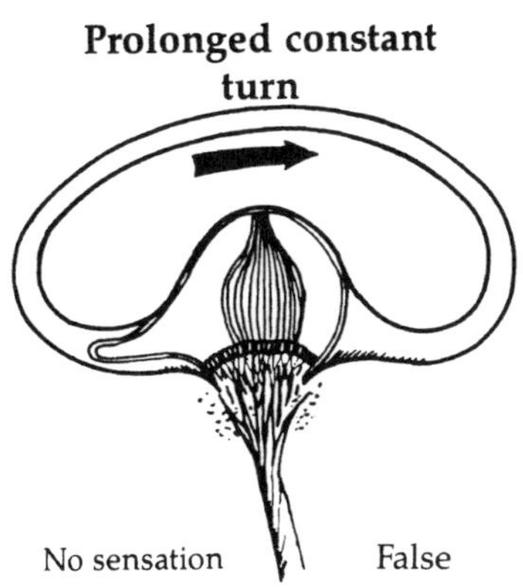

Hair cell position and resulting sensation under conditions of prolonged constant turn.

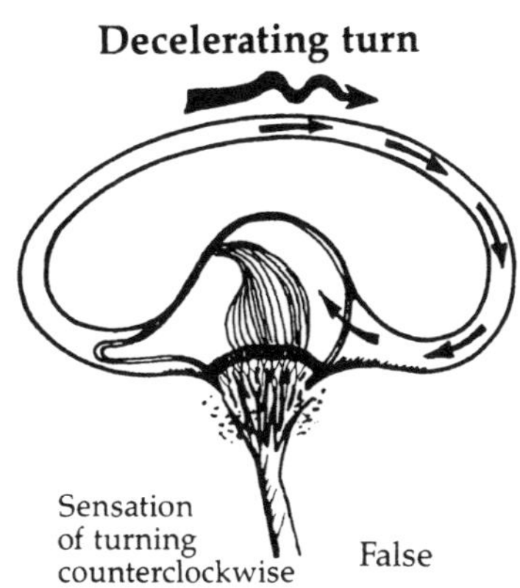

Hair cell position and resulting sensation under conditions of sudden stop or slowing.

hair cells move in the same way that sea grass moves with the water currents and wheat fields move in the wind. As the currents and winds change, so does the movement of the plants.) This movement in turn stimulates the vestibular nerve and impulses are transmitted to your brain where they are interpreted as rotation of your head.

When no acceleration takes place, the hair cells do not move and remain upright and a sense of "no turn" is felt. When a semicircular canal is put into motion, as during the acceleration of a turn or in ascent or descent, the fluid within the canals moves, but there is a lag in the response along the canal walls because the hair cells bend in the direction opposite to that of the acceleration. The brain interprets the movement of the hairs as motion, or a turn.

Vestibular Illusions

The vestibular system, along with other sources of orienting sensations, works well in keeping you balanced with the rest of

Fig. 3-4 Forward acceleration in an aircraft tricks the hair cells into perceiving a false sensation of tilting backward.

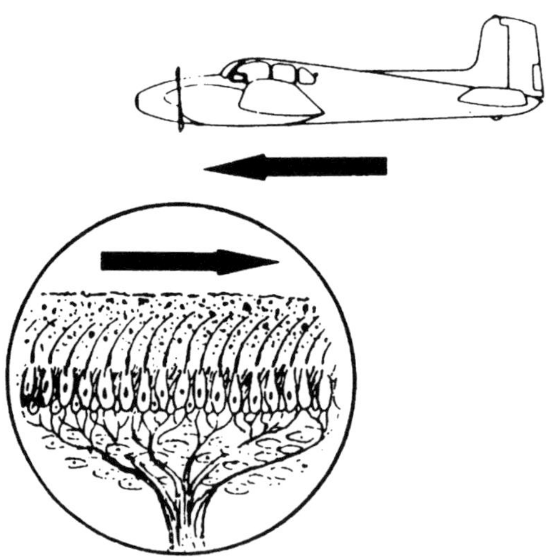

False sensation of backward tilt

the world (Fig. 3-4). When you are subjected to the variables of flight's different forces on your body, however, these orienting sources do not function the way your body and mind is used to and give you misleading information.

Coriolis: Coriolis, another name for vestibular disorientation, is the most dangerous illusion because of its often overwhelming sense of disorientation, and it can occur in any phase of flight where some type of climbing or descending turn is initiated. In discussing weather, coriolus is the effect on wind as it passes over a rotating earth. In physiology it represents the tumbling of your internal gyros or the semicircular canals (Fig. 3-5). Some pilots describe the sensation as being like a giant hand taking over their instruments, fighting their urge to move the stick.

When you and your airplane are straight and level and without acceleration, the fluid in your semicircular canals is in equilibrium (it is not moving). When your aircraft turns and

Fig. 3-5. If a pilot moves his or her head abruptly during a prolonged turn, the coriolis effect can cause an overwhelming illusion of change of aircraft altitude.

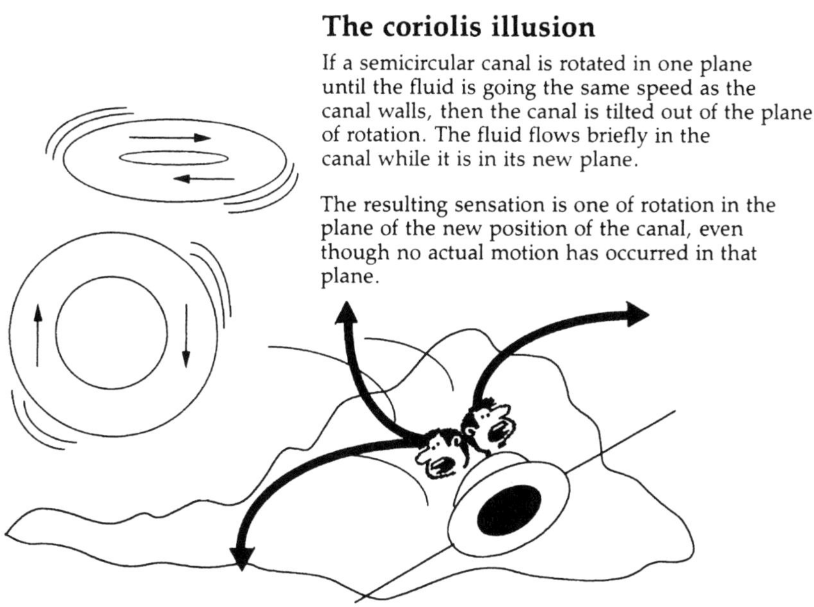

banks, however, there is an accelerative force on the fluid that tells you there is a change. If you stay in that turn, the fluid once again reaches equilibrium and does not move. Thus, only when there is change does the fluid move and give out a signal to the brain. All three positional planes of the canals are affected to varying degrees during a turn, depending on the rate and degree of turn.

If the turn is coordinated and not abrupt, there is minimal misinformation going to your brain. If, however, during a maneuver of a turn, you should turn your head in a different direction from the turn, such as downward, one of these planes is disrupted (tumbled) and sends a misleading cue to the brain as if the plane was in a roll or yaw. The coriolis illusion makes you perceive your aircraft to be doing maneuvers that it is not actually doing. This illusion also can be induced in turbulence during a climb or descending turn. It's the sudden and subtle change to the vestibular apparatus that causes this illusion.

Without a visual reference to the horizon, this illusion can overpower your recognized need to recover, creating a conflict between the sensation expected in the maneuver and the requirement to control the aircraft against that sensation. It is easier to demonstrate this illusion than describe it and this is why unusual attitudes are practiced in flight and why it is recommended that a ride in a Vertigon-type simulator (a device that demonstrates coriolis or vestibular disorientation) be experienced. Flight simulators exploit these signals to mimic aircraft motion without actually moving like the plane.

Leans: This is the most common illusion and occurs when you sense a bank angle when the aircraft is actually in level flight. (Fig. 3-6). If you maintain the level attitude of the aircraft (as you should), you still feel compelled to align your body with the perceived vertical. In doing so, you actually lean in the opposite direction of the perceived turn.

The leans can easily occur if your attention is removed from the instruments for even a short period of time. For example, if during this distraction your aircraft begins to turn slowly to the right, undetected by you, the canals respond accordingly. After a period of time in the turn, your brain forgets that it is in a

Fig. 3-6 The leans.

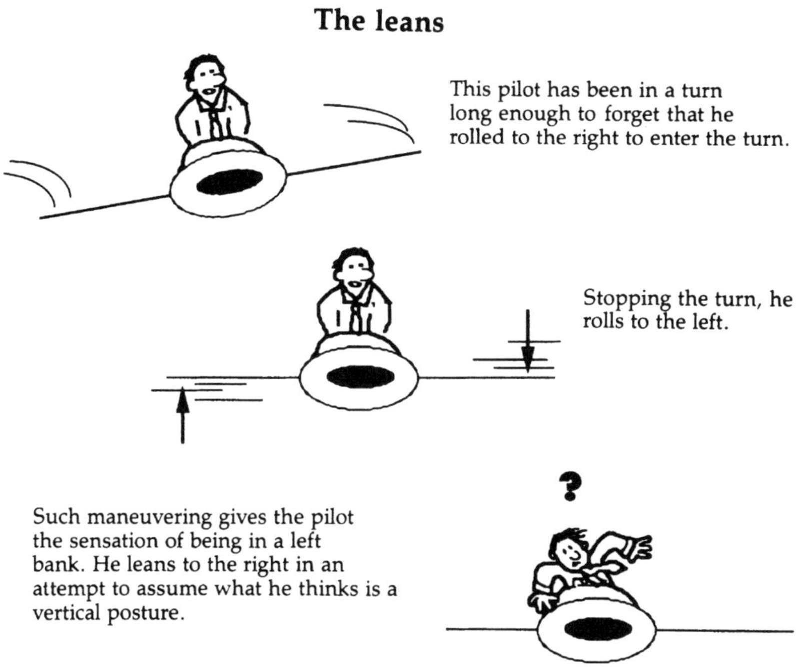

turn. When your attention is directed back to the aircraft and instruments and you return to level flight, you have a false sense that the aircraft is banking to the left. If you react to your senses rather than to the instruments, especially in IMC, you will roll your aircraft to the right.

Oculogravic Illusion: When your aircraft accelerates or decelerates in level flight, your otolith organs sense a nose-high attitude relative to gravity (Fig. 3-7). If you react to this sensation without cross-checking instruments, you may pitch the aircraft down to correct the perception. Deceleration causes a sensation of a nose-low attitude.

Rotational Illusion: In *rotational illusion*, also called *angular motion illusion*, rotational symptoms result from misinformation

Fig. 3-7 Oculogravic illusion.

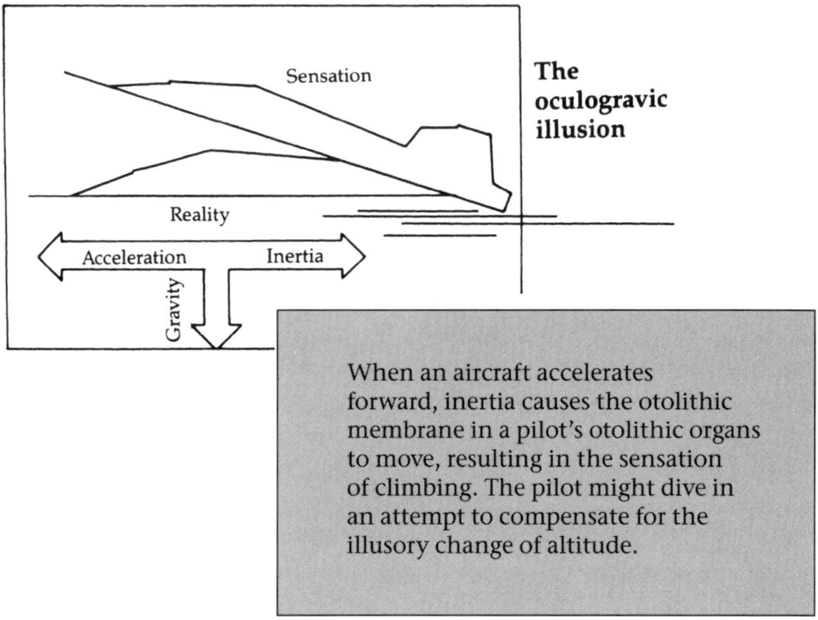

from a constant rate turn, as in a spin. If the turn is at a constant rate, the fluid in the canals returns to equilibrium. This results in your perception that the turn has stopped. When the turn slows (a change as in acceleration) or your aircraft levels off, the fluid is once again displaced but this time in the opposite direction.

The graveyard spin is a condition most likely to affect fixed-wing aircraft pilots (Fig. 3-8). Upon recovering from the turn (or spin) as just described, you undergo deceleration, which will be sensed by your semicircular canals and interpreted as a spin or turn in the opposite direction. Your instruments tell you that you are not spinning but you have a strong sensation that you are spinning. If there is no outside reference to the horizon and you disregard or don't believe the instruments, you are tempted to make control corrections against the falsely perceived spin so that you reenter a spin in the original direction.

This action is compounded by you noting a loss of altitude

as the spin develops and you may apply back pressure on the controls and add power in an attempt to gain altitude. These responses tighten the spin to the point where recovery is nearly impossible.

Fig. 3-8 A graveyard spin illusion is a type of rotational illusion that is most likely to affect fixed-wing pilots.

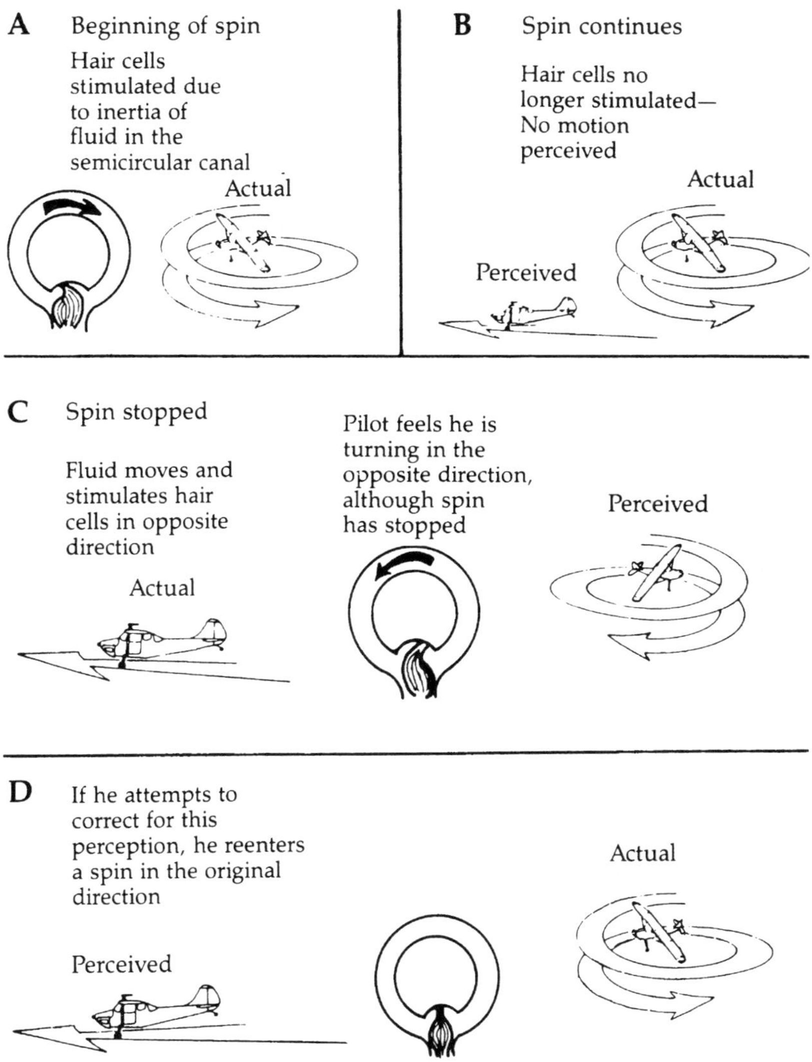

Spatial Disorientation

Spatial disorientation defines illusions associated with relative motion, often called *vection illusion*. Furthermore, spatial infers a visual orientation: how you are oriented to the horizon as straight and level, in a turn, or climbing or descending. Spatial disorientation differs from vestibular disorientation or coriolis.

Of all the senses available to provide input to your brain, vision provides the most valuable information. As much as 90 percent of the usable cues for orientation may come from vision. Your visual acuity comes from your central vision (foveal). Your peripheral vision (ambient) supports your perceived position in space. This peripheral vision is so strong in relaying your body position to the brain that it is estimated that 90 percent of visual sensation on orientation is from peripheral vision. You can see the potential conflict in instrument conditions, in which central vision is used to read your instruments and virtually no peripheral vision exists to establish spatial orientation.

Because peripheral vision is a powerful source of determining balance and orientation, it should be easy to understand why everyone experiences spatial disorientation, whether in a car or in an airplane. Looking straight ahead and concentrating on where you are going or scanning instruments maintains direction. Out of the corner of your eye, observe some visible objects, such as another airplane next to you on the ramp slowly moving, or flying through snow or rain, and you will feel the effects.

Treatment of Spatial Disorientation

- Get on the instruments and develop a good cross-check.
- Never try to fly both VFR and IFR at the same time.
- Delay intuitive actions long enough to check both visual references and your instruments.
- Transfer control if there are two pilots in the aircraft. Seldom will two pilots experience disorientation at the same time.

For example, while sitting at an intersection in your car, waiting for the light to turn green, you suddenly perceive your car moving backward. You slam on your breaks only to realize your car is stationary. It's the car next to you, creeping forward in anticipation of the traffic light, that confused you. Your peripheral vision was telling you how to react with the relative motion of the two cars.

For helicopter pilots, the same illusion is apparent when hovering over tall grass, for example. The wave action of the moving grass gives you the sensation of moving when in fact you are not. Flying in clouds with strobe and other anticollision lights generates the same confusing cues.

Instability varies depending on many conditions. One of the intents of maintaining flying currency is to be able to suppress inputs from your peripheral vision and increase dependency on your central vision. Unfamiliarity of the aircraft also increases vulnerability to your peripheral vision cues.

Spatial disorientation, as described, becomes a serious source of disorientation, especially in instrument conditions. If you are physiologically impaired (tired, hypoxic, using over-the-counter [OTC] drugs, etc.) you lose your tolerance to suppressing inputs from your peripheral vision. You can quickly become incapacitated as a result of conflicting spatial senses.

Visual Illusions in Flight

Visual illusions affect what you perceive through vision, which in turn determines how you respond. It is more of a misguidance in a flying activity (such as landing and judging distances), as opposed to the illusions of disorientation, wherein your body automatically responds to physiological cues from your vestibular system and peripheral vision. They are obviously related in that they both can lead to incapacitation, especially when the events occur concurrently.

Autokinesis

Autokinesis is the perception of false movement when you look at a static source of light for a period of time (minutes) in the dark (Fig. 3-9). This reference point misperceived as moving (an actual illusion) could lead you to follow it. Prevention

Fig. 3-9 To a pilot suffering from autokinesis illusion, a static light, stared at for several seconds, appears to move.

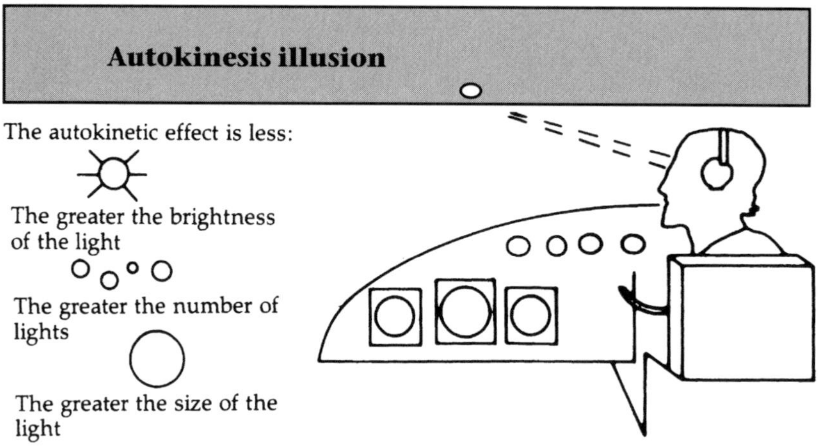

is a combination of realizing the eye must focus on other objects at varying distances, and not fixate on the target, plus applying basic scanning techniques.

Oculogyral

Oculogyral illusions were previously described under physiological disorientation. From the visual point of view, this illusion is more apparent at night, when vision is already compromised. You perceive the apparent movement of an object in the visual field as a result of stimulation of your semicircular canals. Therefore, in the early stages of a turn to the left, for example, the target appears to move rapidly to the left. After the turn is established and then stopped, the target object appears to move in the opposite direction, or to the right. You may correct your aircraft accordingly unless you scan your instruments and confirm that you are tracking an illusion.

Oculogravic

Oculogravic illusion, also called *somatogravic illusion*, is a perception of tilt induced by stimulation of your otolith organs, as previously described in disorientation. From the visual perspective, the illusion to you is either a climb or descent when you have no visual reference to the horizon. With a climb, your eyes try to compensate with a downward tracking, as is common when flying through an updraft. This illusion is also called an *elevator illusion*. The opposite illusion, familiar in helicopter flight, in an autorotation, is the intuitive response of the pilot to change direction and or altitude, which can decrease airspeed below a desired level.

Visual Cue Illusions

There are also illusions that are strictly visual and that mislead you into erroneous actions. This type of illusion is not a physiological event associated with the semicircular canals; it is the interpretation of your brain of an image as a result of the illusion of misleading visual cues. The greatest chance of these illusions affecting flight is in the landing phase and, to a lesser degree, in cruise where outside visual cues can be misleading.

Fog and Haze

Depth perception, or the ability of your brain to determine relative distance from visual cues, is compromised by any atmospheric conditions that interfere with light transmission. In addition to obscuring the ground and nearby outside obstacles, fog and haze refract light rays differently than clear air, leading to out-of-focus acuity. Contrast is reduced, which is important in defining size and shape. It becomes difficult for you to judge distances, especially height above ground and distance from the end of the runway. Light from ground lights, including REILs, VASI, runway and taxiway lights, is diffused, losing the detail necessary for a precision approach and landing. Penetration into fog can create the illusion of pitching up.

Water Refraction

Rain on the windshield refracts incoming light rays, which misleads you concerning the position of the horizon, thus, the perception is that the horizon is below where it actually is, especially on an approach, resulting in a lower approach.

Landing Visual Illusions

Runway width that is narrower than usual or expected tends to make you think you are higher than you actually are and you fly a lower approach. A greater width than expected has the opposite effect; thus, the approach being too high.

An up-sloping runway or surrounding terrain can result in the illusion that your aircraft is higher (the glide path appears high) than in actuality, resulting in a lower approach. Down-sloping runways produce the opposite result: The glide path appears low and the approach may be high.

The absence of ground features such as buildings and trees with which you can relate distance can cause you to think you are higher in the air. Flying an approach over water at night, for example, without frequent referral to instruments results in a lower approach height—the black hole effect.

Recognizing the importance of peripheral and central vision inputs to your brain, it should be respected that visual cues can be disorienting in addition to misleading you in your position. It should be obvious that the scan and cross-check of instruments become a critical part of any flight activity. Only practice and currency overcomes these illusions.

Coping with Disorientation

If a healthy pilot can become disoriented and visual illusions affect everyone, then a less-than-healthy pilot is at greater risk. Any one or a combination of the following conditions degrades your performance, especially during critical phases of flight.

The following conditions are each discussed in subsequent chapters and are identified here to raise the level of awareness of their importance. Conditions that can reduce your tolerance to overcoming the effects described previously include the use of alcohol (even hours before flight), hypoglycemia, fatigue, use of medication, illness, and hypoxia. If you suffer from any of these conditions, you must be particularly careful about instrument scans, attentive to all communications, and maintain a high level of awareness and cross-checking to monitor performance.

You can cope with these situations of disorientation and illusions by maintaining currency in familiar aircraft. Flight proficiency is absolutely essential. The lack of either reduces your tolerance to these potentially incapacitating events. Every pilot knows that he or she becomes rusty in performance skills, often after only a few days of nonflying. Flying instruments only once in awhile puts you at high risk of unacceptable performance when eventful instrument conditions arise. There is no substitute for training and maintaining currency.

Flicker Vertigo

Flicker vertigo is a poorly understood sensation, and is probably not as serious or as frequent as one would expect. Some pilots, especially in helicopters, suffer a variety of symptoms from light that has a strobelike flashing or flickering to the eyes. This effect occurs as light from the sun or other source is reflected off a propeller or rotor blades or is interrupted in the same cycle by the props. The rate is about 4 to 20 cycles per second and can produce unpleasant and potentially dangerous reactions. Nausea, vomiting, and fatigue can result. In extreme cases in highly susceptible pilots, neurological reactions may occur such as convulsions and changes in levels of consciousness. A pilot who suffers from the previously mentioned conditions is also at higher risk. There is a great deal of anecdotal information, but little scientific data, to confirm an actual flicker vertigo.

The Airsick Pilot

The vestibular system appears to be the source of the symptoms of motion sickness (airsickness). Any pilot, subjected to the right combination of unusual attitudes or flight conditions, can become airsick. Thus, if the semicircular canals can be tumbled in a way to which you are not adapted, then you become sick. There is no doubt that familiarity with the aircraft and its typical maneuvers, currency, and self-confidence is the best deterrent to airsickness.

Passengers (or pilots not in control of the aircraft) are easy victims of airsickness. New pilots are also susceptible. Some additional, common causes of airsickness include heat discomfort, anxiety, observing or smelling someone else who is airsick, and eating foods that are nauseating.

With full motion and full visual field simulators, there is increasing awareness of a condition called *simulator sickness*. The motions of such simulators do not mimic the actual motions of an aircraft. For example, when the sensation of climb is noted, the simulator is not pointing upward; rather, there are clever motions of the simulator that fool the vestibular system into perceiving a climb. Couple this perception with that from your peripheral vision and you can duplicate an amazing sense of reality. Worse, if the visual portion of the simulator is a fraction of a second off the actual physical motion, airsickness can occur. Of greater significance is the development of ataxia (unsteady gait) after being in a simulator for several hours. It's advised that a pilot delay driving or flying for a few hours to ensure there is no aftereffect.

Most people know if they are prone to airsickness . Even so, there is no known dependable prevention technique or adequate treatment to help with this condition. Research is being carried out because motion sickness is a prime concern in space travel. Some suggest that there is more chance of becoming airsick if you fly on an empty stomach. Therefore, before you fly you should eat simple foods that you know you can tolerate, including adequate fluids. There are a variety of medications available, both OTC and prescribed. There is little reliability or predictability from one person to another, however, in their effectiveness and there are often unsafe side effects of the common drugs.

Flying in Heat and Cold Extremes 4

It was a balmy 72°F February day when our U.S. Air Force crew left Kansas for a 5-day trip to Alaska. The reality of where we were hit us square in the face when we opened the hatch upon landing and experienced −50°F, which was the actual temperature, with no windchill added. After unloading our gear, I sat in the cockpit while the aircraft was towed (power off). It was the worst 15 minutes I had ever spent in a cockpit. My body began to shiver almost uncontrollably. I couldn't move switches because I couldn't grab them. My mental and physical activity slowed down and I tried to move as little as possible. When finally in my hotel room, I recalled the exhaustion I had experienced during those 15 minutes. I could hardly get my winter clothing off. On the return trip, we were in such a scramble to get through the preflight and get airborne that after takeoff I noticed that the fuel panel switches had been improperly positioned, all because we had rushed.

THERE ARE FEW PLACES on earth that have a constant type of weather system. Temperatures, winds, dew points (humidity), and rain are continually changing. Some parts of the world have weather extremes that last for months, allowing inhabitants to acclimate to the season. Those of you living and flying in the northern latitudes of the northern hemisphere adapt to cold winters, whereas those of you living in the hot humid areas find the conditions in the north during winter not only unbearable but also dangerous.

Your body and mind have the metabolic resources to respond to these weather variations and extremes, which allows you to continue to perform. Sometimes, however, your body may react in adverse ways that interfere with expected performance, again, both physically and mentally. This interference equates to impairment of your piloting skills, making you less than safe and, in effect, incapacitated.

Modern flying machines take us great distances, not only within our own country but also around the world, all in a matter of a few hours to 1 or 2 days. Therefore, as the pilot of these machines or the flight attendant in the cabin, you are exposed to variations of extremes of weather conditions without the advantages of adapting or becoming acclimated. Furthermore, you are often unprepared to cope with these extremes, flying without adequate protective clothing and being in less-than-ideal physical condition. Depending on the aircraft you fly, any time of the year, it may not be uncommon for you to depart from a cold, dry, windy airport and arrive several hours later at a hot, humid, calm destination. And you probably will stay there only a few hours or days before heading back or going on to another location of variable weather extremes.

Basics of Heat Exchange

Because you often resort to basic stick-and-rudder skills during complex situations, let's start our discussion of how the environment impacts your piloting skills by reviewing the basics of temperature extremes. The first thing to realize is that the definition of cold is the absence of heat. Absolute zero temperature (–459.67° F) means there is no heat—no energy. As the energy of heat is added, the temperature rises. Therefore, in any discussion of temperature-related situations, it's important to understand that we are talking mainly about the transfer of heat, not cold.

What happens in your body is essentially the same physics as occurs in your home. Warming up the building means adding heat to the circulating air. Cooling means removing heat. How this heat is exchanged depends on physical properties of heat transfer (Fig. 4-1).

Heat that is transferred by direct contact with another object is called *conduction*. Conduction can occur within the same object, such as an airplane, by going from one part to another (e.g., heat from the engine warming the airframe). The more common situation is when a part of the body, such as your hands or feet, comes in contact with another object that is colder or warmer, perhaps by sitting in a cold seat or leaning

Fig. 4-1 The first law of thermodynamics states that heat is transferred from hotter to colder objects.

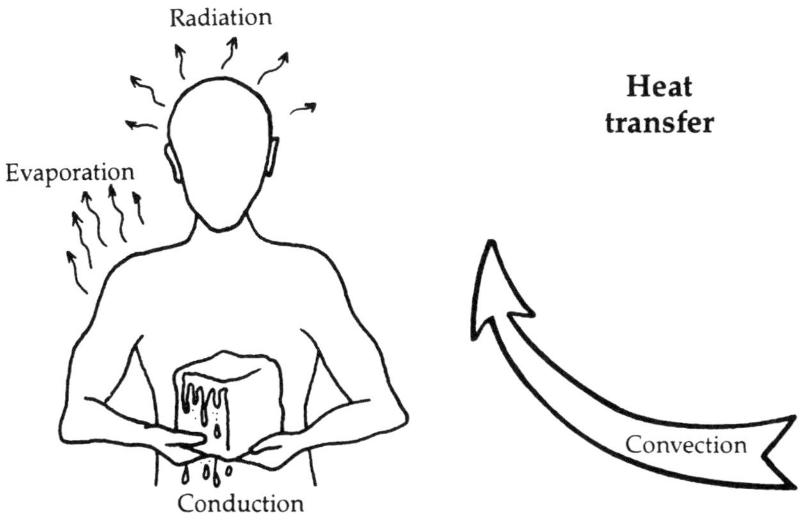

against the wall of an airplane parked on the ramp in the middle of summer.

Convection is the most common way to transfer heat. In convection, heat is moved within gasses or liquids as it flows from one object to another, such as in a building or airplane cabin. Air is heated by a flame or hot object (engine) and the airflow carries this heat to another part of the building or aircraft. You feel warm as the heat is transferred from the air to your skin. Depending on the ambient temperature (the temperature of the surrounding air), the relative flow of air as it moves across your body also becomes a major factor in heat transfer. In addition to wind, this flow can be from a fan or from your body moving in an open cockpit. Even if there is no difference between the temperature of the moving air and your body, you still feel colder because of windchill, described later. Within your body, heat transfer is performed by warm blood carrying heat from one part of the body to another.

When heat is transferred from one object to another of different temperature without being carried by a gas or liquid (and you're not touching anything), it is *radiation*. The transfer is in the form of electromagnetic waves. The sun is the most obvious source of radiation. You often feel the warmth from the sun on your skin even though the ambient temperature is low. The amount of heat transferred depends on the size of the radiating object, the relative difference of temperature, and, like with light, exponentially on the distance from that object. Radiation also initiates the greenhouse effect in a cockpit of an airplane sitting on the ramp in the sun or in your car in the driveway. Grabbing the yoke or wheel on a blistering day quickly familiarizes you with radiation.

Evaporation is another form of heat transfer; it requires energy or heat to change a liquid to a gas. Mechanical refrigeration with a compressor uses this physical property because heat is taken away from the container (refrigerator) as the refrigerant expands. As with machinery, the same holds true with your body. Sweat, for example, evaporates off the skin and in doing so takes heat away from the skin.

How you feel, your level of comfort, also determines how effective you are when performing your job. If you feel too hot or too cold then your performance is substandard. This comfort factor is dependent on all these forms of heat transfer and to varying degrees and combinations. For example, in a small cockpit or small airplane, radiant solar heat warms the air and body without heat from any other source. The greenhouse effect can raise the temperature 10 to 15°C higher without any other heat source. Convected heat (or lack of heat) from air vents and heaters supplements the radiant energy. Sitting in a hot or cold seat conducts heat to or from the body. And if you are sweating from the preflight activities, evaporation adds to the discomfort (or comfort). It's subjective, and each crewmember responds differently and unpredictably.

Temperature Control in the Body

Quick—what is the proper temperature of your body? 98.6°F, 89.6°F, somewhere between the two? If you said 98.6°F, you are on your way to understanding core temperature. The core defines critical organs such as the brain, heart, liver, and lungs.

This core of organs must be kept at a constant temperature (average of 98.6°F) if you are to be kept in good spirits. This distinguishes you as a warm-blooded animal from cold-blooded animals whose core temperatures stay close to ambient temperatures. Failure of warm-blooded animals to keep the core temperature within this range (96.6 to 99.5°F) results in depressed performance and ultimately leads to total incapacitation.

Therefore, the goal of your body's temperature control system is to maintain body core temperature constant, often at the expense of temperature control in other parts and organs of the body. This requires a properly functioning body in good physical condition. Temperature control incorporates all the physics of heat transfer and flow, heat generation, air-(blood) conditioning, and heat and cold regulation.

Heat is the ultimate form of energy and is generated by virtually all activities of your body, but mainly from muscle activity. In fact, it is estimated that so much heat is created that if it weren't dispersed, the core temperature would rise to 190°F! Your body, therefore, has a vast resource of available heat. When heat is needed and not externally available, your body responds by shivering, which is its way of involuntarily increasing muscle activity and more heat. All muscle activity requires internal calories from the energy of ingested food. It follows, therefore, that during periods when heat is needed, more food must be eaten to provide adequate fuel.

The skin is considered a major heat exchange component because of its large surface area, which is conveniently exposed to the outside air for transfer of heat. The more blood that reaches the skin, the more heat that can be dissipated, provided the heat is taken from the skin either by convection or evaporation. The amount of blood reaching the skin is controlled by the ability of the arteries to shunt blood away from or to the skin. Vasodilatation and vasoconstriction of arteries play an important rôle in this process.

In a hot environment, your body must get rid of excessive heat in the core to prevent the core temperature from rising. It does so by opening the arteries to the skin and within the skin, allowing more blood to get to the surface area of your body to dissipate the heat. The skin becomes red and flushed as a result of the superficial blood vessels getting wider (like the blush after a bad landing that can sometimes generate the same effect). The reverse is true in a cold environment. To preserve the core temperature, blood is shunted away from the skin and concentrated in the core, resulting in pale and blanched skin color. This leads to poor warming of the extremities and other outer body parts with the poor blood supply (e.g., nose and ears).

It should be apparent that efficient blood flow is dependent on an efficient circulatory system and a healthy heart. Therefore, those in poor physical condition are less effective at tolerating temperature extremes. Also, self-induced stresses (alcohol, self-medication, dehydration, poor nutrition, etc.) seriously compromise the ability to effectively cope with temperature extremes and reduce effective acclimatization.

Your body can generate heat and shunt excess heat to the surface of the body to be dispelled. Heat removal by radiation and by convection of moving air, however, is not efficient. Heat also has to be taken away from your skin by evaporation of sweat on the skin. Because evaporation requires heat, according to the laws of physics, this process is effective in using the heat in the skin.

Just as additional fuel is needed for generation of heat through increased muscle activity, your body needs more water under conditions of increased sweat production. This need is internal, which means fluids must be available within the body to be effective. Because sweat includes some electrolytes (mainly sodium and potassium chloride), you must be aware of depletion of these electrolytes during high losses of sweat, especially if you are not acclimated to your surroundings.

Anyone who has ever climbed into a cockpit on a hot day wearing a uniform knows that it serves no purpose if sweat doesn't evaporate or the evaporated sweat isn't effectively removed to make room for more sweat to be evaporated. Those of you flying in conditions of high humidity (or dew points), wherein evaporation cannot take place, appreciate how sweat can accumulate. It's a complex situation because enough skin must be exposed for the ambient air to remove the sweat through evaporation, yet there must be protection of the skin to prevent overheating from radiation, conduction, and convection present in the working environment.

Most of what I have discussed so far takes little or no conscious effort on your part to accomplish. Thermoregulatory centers take input from your body's receptors and then generate heat by either increasing muscle activity, which warms the blood, or increasing sweat production, which cools the blood. The centers then regulate the flow of blood between the core and the skin to either conserve heat or dissipate heat to the core. In extreme conditions, some conscious effort must be taken, however, to assist your body's own actions.

In the Heat of Flight: Flying When Hot

It was 95°F when I left home and headed for the airport with every intention of going on a short cross-country in my Bonanza. Things

Apparent Temperature

Since both temperature and humidity act in combination with one another, there's a system for measuring their combined effects on the body. It's called the "heat index" (formerly known as the temperature humidity index).

The heat index (HI) couples the temperature and relative humidity into an "apparent temperature." If, for example, the temperature is 90 degrees fahrenheit and the relative humidity is 65%, the HI, or apparent temperature, would be 102 degrees.

The HI is a more accurate means of gauging the effects of heat and humidity on the body's cooling system. Increasing temperatures cause the body to sweat more, and increasing humidity decreases the air's capacity to absorb the sweat and facilitate cooling.

When the HI is in the 80–90 degree range, fatigue is likely during prolonged activity; when it is in the 90–105 range, sunstroke and heat exhaustion are possible; 105–130 indicates that sunstroke and heat exhaustion are likely; 130 or higher indicates that heatstroke is most likely.

changed rapidly when I arrived at the hangar and remembered I had left the aircraft sitting outside. It had to be 125°F or more inside the cockpit. I couldn't do a preflight because there was so much sweat running in my eyes, and I couldn't read the dials. What was meant to be a pleasure trip had turned into a miserable experience and not such a hot idea (no pun intended). I was in the cockpit for maybe 10 minutes and I was already soaking wet. I decided to push the aircraft in the hangar and wait for another day.

As mentioned earlier, when your body's thermoregulatory center senses that the core temperature is increasing, certain functions begin to take place. Blood supply is shunted to the core where heat is accumulating. The heated blood is quickly taken to the skin where the dilated blood vessels warm the skin relative to the amount of heat being dissipated. As in the example above, the more heat, the higher the skin temperature. Concurrently, sweat volume is increased from the sweat glands for evaporation. If you stay in this hot environment too long, as much as 4 to 16 quarts of water can be lost through sweating and respiration, especially if you are active.

Obviously, this fluid must be replaced. From a comfort point of view, a crewmember, given enough water, can function all day at a temperature of 115°F with a relative humidity of 10%. If, however, the relative humidity is raised to 80%, this same person can be incapacitated within 30 minutes. Dew point is sometimes a better indicator of anticipated discomfort. If it is above 60°F with the outside air temperature at any level above this, you will be uncomfortable, which could be as disabling as the physiological conditions to be discussed later.

Some of the conditions that make you less tolerant to heat extremes include increasing age, excessive alcohol intake (alcohol dilates blood vessel and prevents efficient shunting), lack of sleep, obesity, and previous history of heat stroke (the more serious kind of heat stress). Lack of being adequately acclimated makes you much more susceptible.

General Symptoms of Heat Stress

As your body temperature increases (hyperthermia) and struggles to maintain a constant core temperature, there are some symptoms that have a direct effect on your piloting performance. These symptoms include less reliable short-term memory, an increase in error rate, erosion of motor skills, and a general decrease in performance skill. Heat stress increases your irritability and diminishes insight into judgment skills, creating a tendency to overreact and make more mistakes. Heat also increases the susceptibility to motion sickness, hypoxia, and any degree of G forces. In addition, fatigue becomes apparent after several hours of coping with heat.

Specific Heat Stresses

In addition to the previously mentioned generalized symptoms, the following are physiological stages of heat stress that need to be recognized. As each stage evolves without recognition and treatment intervention, you become increasingly impaired to the point of becoming completely incapacitated.

Heat Cramps

Heat cramps, also called minor heat stress, occur when body temperature of 99.5 to 100.5°F is reached. Painful muscle cramps of the extremities, abdomen, and back are common in heat. Heat cramps are an indicator of the early stage of fluid depletion. Identification of this stage is important because this is when the body's struggle to maintain its own temperature control is occurring. Treatment consists of rest, getting out of the heat and into shade, and forcing fluids as much as can be tolerated. Drinking water is all that's necessary.

Heat Exhaustion

In heat exhaustion, body temperature can reach 101 to 105°F. Heat exhaustion represents the first serious stage where your body begins to be unable to keep up with controlling core temperature. The thermoregulatory system is still working and the body is responding with proper shunting of blood and enough sweat to evaporate; however, if the conditions are severe with high heat, high dew points, little or no shade, high activity levels, and no wind, the body is unable to keep up without rest and more fluids. Outside conditions play a crucial role in determining the severity of this stage.

Symptoms of heat exhaustion include headache, confusion, incoordination, loss of appetite, nausea, and cramps (not to be confused with a hangover). Because your heat control system is still functioning, you sweat, which means the skin is moist and still relatively cool. But the cardiovascular system is working harder to keep up with the increased heart rate necessary to overcome the dilated vessels during the transport of heat from blood flow.

The treatment for heat exhaustion is to get out of the heat and help your body's heat exchange processes function. Rest in the shade or in a cooler setting is mandatory. Fluids are especially important. Ingesting water is probably all that is needed at this stage. Do not be overly concerned about salt replacement; there's usually plenty of salt in the food you eat. You cannot take in too much water because the kidneys get rid of any excess. Too much water intake, however, can cause nausea and vomiting when ingested too quickly. Continual sipping of cool water is ideal.

A key point is that if you are ever in this condition, you have reached the limits of your body's attempt to control core temperature. You are "behind the power curve." Therefore, returning to work or to flying is not safe for several hours.

Heat Stroke

If you are experiencing heat stroke, your body temperature is above 105°F. Heat stroke is the last phase of inadequate temperature control and the most serious. It is a medical emergency when identified. Your body is no longer capable of defending itself because the thermoregulatory system has broken down and is unable to control the body temperature control functions and keep core temperature acceptable. You'll find yourself already significantly impaired and may become unconscious in a short time.

The key to heat stroke diagnosis is the lack of any body cooling activity. Sweat is no longer being produced and therefore there is no evaporation taking place. The skin is dry and hot. The core temperature may reach as high as 106°F, which is life-threatening.

The first step is to get to a cool place. Treatment includes calling for medical assistance to get fluids into the body intra-

Heat Stroke

Causes:

- High temperature and high humidity
- Changes in climate
- Inadequate solar protection
- Exertion
- Past incidence of heat stroke
- Dehydration
- Medication (certain drugs interfere with perspiration)
- Illness
- Skin problems

Prevention:

- WATER!

venously, along with any methods to cool the body down, such as immersion in cool water, and spraying or pouring any liquid over the body to help cooling by evaporation.

In general, when in hot conditions, whether on the ground or in the air, be suspicious of extreme conditions and look for potential heat-induced symptoms in others as well as in yourself.

Prevention

As with any other medical problem, prevention is the best cure. Heat stress could be considered self-induced because you have control of prevention. The most important part of prevention is drinking more than enough fluids. That means drinking water before subjecting yourself to heat extremes. Maintaining hydration is the single most important goal. In hot weather, an average person requires 2 or 3 gallons of fluid per day in addition to that supplied in a normal meal. If taken internally, fluids do you more good than if they are poured over the outside of the body. The latter may make you feel cooler but your body's heat control system needs ingested water to replace evaporated sweat. Thirst is a poor indicator of need because you are already dehydrated when you are thirsty. The ideal prevention is to always carry a large plastic container, especially the one with a built-in sipping straw, filled with water and continually sip from it.

Avoid fluids known to contain diuretics, such as caffeine and alcohol, especially prior to being subjected to heat extremes. (A diuretic is a chemical that increases the production of urine.) Tea, as in ice tea, is particularly bad because there are two diuretics present—caffeine and theophyline. If you are not acclimated to the environment, salt may be added to food but salt tablets are not generally required. Most Americans (pilots and flight attendants included) consume more salt than is considered healthy.

Protective clothing is important, provided it still allows for circulation of air over the skin. White, loose, lightweight clothing is preferable. Protection of the head is also important to shield the skull from a heat load.

It may seem overstated to consider heat stress a problem to aircrew who are in flight. Consider, however, that you also may spend a lot of time out of the airplane, such as during preflight and loading, on a hot ramp in humid weather. You may be dehydrated before showing up for the flight. If you then jump into the hot aircraft, already low on fluids, your body continues to be heat stressed with the same symptoms as if you were still outside. After sitting in a hot cockpit as a result of the greenhouse effect, it could take more than 20 minutes just to recover after the cabin finally cools.

Prior to acclimatization, your capacity to work in heat or cold is impaired. Your body senses the changes in climate and adjusts its thermoregulatory system, which alerts the body to prepare for more efficient use of body fluids and heat generation. Essentially, your body makes diluted sweat in hot environments and more of it, sooner. Subjectively, you cope better in hot environments and can be more active both physically and mentally without undue impairment.

It takes 2 or 3 weeks to completely adjust to a new environment. Therefore, if you live in a climate that turns cool in the fall and travel to a hot humid location for a few days, you will not become acclimated in that amount of time and therefore are at high risk of developing heat stress. Conversely, living in warm climates and trying to cope in below-freezing conditions is equally as impairing.

Frigid Air: Flying When Cold

Have you ever preflighted your aircraft on a really cold day? It's been said that the length of the preflight in cold conditions is directly proportional to the temperature. Cold extremes can be incapacitating. Coping with the cold basically involves generating and conserving heat. Enough heat is generated by your body if you are active and have enough caloric fuel. The primary goal, then, is to protect your body from losing too much of the heat that is already present.

Hypothermia Symptoms

In the early stages of hypothermia (exposure), there is obvious discomfort leading to distraction. As you get colder, you may experience muscle stiffness and weakness, fatigue and sometimes drowsiness. Thought processes are dulled and stuporous. As the cold increases, you begin to shiver uncontrollably. These early symptoms are the first signs of clinical hypothermia and corrective action must be taken. As heat is taken away from the core (by the futile attempts of the body's heat conservation system plus the loss of heat from lack of protection of the surface of the body), your body begins to become generally impaired, and you are unable to "keep up." It's just the opposite of trying to keep the body's core cool.

The same heat transfer process is taking place. To conserve heat, blood flow is shunted *away* from the surface at the expense of the extremities and other nonessential body parts. Muscle activity is increased involuntarily. As your body loses this battle, the core temperature continues to decrease.

Hypothermia symptoms are less subtle than with hyperthermia, and in most situations, are more easily controlled, if you are prepared. The degree of heat loss is dependent on your physical condition, the environmental conditions (e.g., temperature and wind), and the protection of your body, especially the large surface area of your skin.

Loss of Body Heat

All the physical properties of heat transfer are in effect in cold extremes, but with variations from those associated with heat. Radiation now becomes the leading cause of heat loss through any uncovered skin. The scalp is especially vulnerable because of its highly vascular anatomy (that's why there is so much bleeding when you get a laceration of the scalp). Hats, therefore, are an essential piece of cold weather clothing.

Conduction is also important if you are in contact with cold seats and instruments and other unheated objects. Wet, cold clothing can remove heat 25 times more rapidly from the body than dry clothing. Sweat soaks the clothing next to your skin. This exposed moisture is cooling as it evaporates, resulting in heat loss from the body first through conduction then convection. Loose clothing is therefore important. Even more important is the layered look, wearing several layers of clothes (pants, sweaters or coats, gloves, hats, etc.) that can be removed or added as comfort levels change. Thus, if you know you are going to be subjected to extremes, it's better to carry a bag of extra clothes than leave them in the office. A hat, gloves, socks, and sweater don't take up much room.

Convection plays a major role in heat loss, especially when surrounded by cold air or cold water. When cold air passes over exposed skin, heat is lost rapidly. This is called *windchill* and it is the product of temperature and wind velocity (Fig. 4-2). Not only is heat lost in a short period of time but also local areas of exposed skin on the extremities and other locations where blood has been shunted away (e.g., ears and nose) will freeze. Any liquid can cause the same problem, including aviation fuel.

Treatment should be obvious. Get out of the cold and immediately remove wet and cold clothing and begin rapid warming of the body (hot bath or shower). Drinking hot beverages also helps. Put on warm clothes and try to maintain some muscle activity.

Fig. 4-2 Windchill is the product of temperature and wind velocity.

WIND SPEED		TEMPERATURE (°F)																						
CALM	CALM	40	35	30	25	20	15	10	5	0	-5	-10	-15	-20	-25	-30	-35	-40	-45	-50	-55	-60
KNOTS	MPH	EQUIVALENT CHILL TEMPERATURE																				
3-6	5	35	30	25	20	15	10	5	0	-5	-10	-15	-20	-25	-30	-35	-40	-45	-50	-55	-65	-70
7-10	10	30	20	15	10	5	0	-10	-15	-20	-25	-35	-40	-45	-50	-60	-65	-70	-75	-80	-90	-95
11-15	15	25	15	10	0	-5	-10	-20	-25	-30	-40	-45	-50	-60	-65	-70	-80	-85	-90	-100	-105	-110
16-19	20	20	10	5	0	-10	-15	-25	-30	-35	-45	-50	-60	-65	-75	-80	-85	-95	-100	-110	-115	-120
20-23	25	15	10	0	-5	-15	-20	-30	-35	-45	-50	-60	-65	-75	-80	-90	-95	-105	-110	-120	-125	-135
24-28	30	10	5	0	-10	-20	-25	-30	-40	-50	-55	-65	-70	-80	-85	-95	-100	-110	-115	-125	-130	-140
29-32	35	10	5	-5	-10	-20	-30	-35	-40	-50	-60	-65	-75	-80	-90	-100	-105	-115	-120	-130	-135	-145
33-36	40	10	0	-5	-15	-20	-30	-35	-45	-55	-60	-70	-75	-85	-95	-100	-110	-115	-125	-130	-140	-150
WINDS ABOVE 40 HAVE LITTLE ADDITIONAL EFFECT.		LITTLE DANGER					INCREASING DANGER (Flesh may freeze within1 minute)						GREAT DANGER (Flesh may freeze within 30 seconds)									
		DANGER OF FREEZING EXPOSED FLESH FOR PROPERLY CLOTHED PERSONS																				

Frostbite

Frostbite is an extreme condition of heat loss from a local area. Tissues are actually frozen and the degree of injury is related to the depth of the freezing. Tissues that are frozen die as a result of the crystallization of tissue and cellular fluids.

The symptoms of frostbite vary. The first sensation is numbness but not pain. Grayish or white spots may show up on the skin before freezing actually occurs. After awhile there is no feeling in the affected area and the tissues are hard to the touch. All this occurs because there has been no internal warming by the blood that has been shunted to the core.

Frostbite to fingers and toes is common in pilots who are on the ramp in slush and spilled fuel. Doing a preflight without gloves, a hat, or other additional protection, excluding your uniform, exposes other areas of your body to risk of frostbite or hypothermia.

Treatment for frostbite includes immediate warming. Do not rub the affected area with snow! Ideally, the affected parts should be immersed in water that is warm to the touch. Be advised that as the tissues thaw, the pain becomes severe. This is not an indication to stop warming. However, if the injury is this severe, medical attention should be obtained.

Prevention of Cold Stress

As with heat stress, prevention is the most important action you can take against cold stress. Not only prevention, through awareness of keeping warm and preventing heat loss, but in preparedness, by having access to and wearing adequate cold-weather clothing when you know you are going to a colder destination.

The specific and obvious measures to follow are to be aware of the temperatures, winds, and windchills at your present location and at the various destinations to which you will be going. Limit the amount of time of exposure, keep your body and clothes dry. If you're sweating and spill water or fuel on your clothes, take them off and put on dry clothes. Use the layered look, wearing several layers of loose clothing that can be removed or added as comfort levels change. Keep your activities below the sweating level.

Alcohol is a vasodilator and thus may make you feel warm (and flushed) because it keeps surface blood vessels wide open. This effect is, however, just the opposite of what your body is trying to do, which is to shunt blood away from the skin. Proper nutrition is equally important if you will be encountering cold conditions. Your body needs calories to generate heat. This means eating high-calorie meals.

Dehydration

Dehydration is very common among aircrew and is not just related to temperature extremes. The lifestyle of the traveling pilot or flight attendant, along with the cockpit and cabin environment, lend themselves to increased risk of becoming dehydrated. Hours of increased dehydration is one reason why kidney stones are relatively common in pilots who fly great distances in a dehydrated condition and who are sedentary for long periods.

Why is dehydration so common in pilots? Because most pilots are not drinking water en route. More often than not, coffee is the fluid of choice, although the trend is toward decaffeinated coffee. Drinking ice tea is counterproductive because it is a strong diuretic. The dilemma is that ice tea is often used as a refreshing beverage in hot environments. Pressurized cockpit humidity approaches less than 10% 20 to 30 minutes after takeoff. Even if the pilot is physically inactive during flight, there is an insensible water loss from respiration and skin of 1,200 milliliters of water per day in ideal conditions, and more so in dry conditions. Flight attendants, who are more active than pilots, can lose even more water.

Consuming a lot of coffee (or tea, including iced tea) before the flight and urinating more liquid than you consumed is another problem. Your level of dehydration, by the way, can be monitored by observing the color of urine: The darker the urine the more you are dehydrated.

Dehydration (for any reason) has similar symptoms to those experienced with heat stress. Common symptoms include headache, dizziness, and especially fatigue, and these symptoms occur in varying stages, from mild to incapacitating. Unfortunately, crewmembers tend to wait for symptoms instead of practicing the commonsense approach of prevention. Thirst is an indicator, but as noted, only after you are already dehydrated.

Radiation

Radiation comes in many forms and each form has a different effect on the body (Fig. 4-3).

Various portions of ultraviolet (UV) light or radiation wavelengths can affect your eyes, specifically the cornea (UVB, 200 to 315 nm), lens (UVA, 315 to 400 nm), and to an uncommon degree, the retina (UVC, 400 to 700). Most UV radiation from the sun is filtered out by the ozone layer in the atmosphere, especially UVC waves. There appears to be increasing evidence, but little proof, that the ozone layer is being depleted. This could increase the risk, especially to pilots flying at high altitudes for long trips, of UV radiation damage. This damage is limited to eye changes, such as cataracts. This is easily prevented by ensuring that all correcting glasses and sunglasses have a UV coating that filters out the UV radiation. It is important that the full UV range (200 to 400 nm) is filtered out. Check the label on the glasses.

Exposure to UV radiation also affects the skin, resulting in the all-too-common sunburn. The UVB causes most of the damage but studies now show that UVA (used in tanning booths) adds to the effect of UVB but it is not as severe as UVB. Few pilots or flight attendants have avoided the symptoms of sunburn and most can remember that a good burn is certainly disabling, and at best distracting. Despite increasing evidence about the relationship between UV radiation and sunburn with skin cancer, tanning still is a summer ritual for some. You can acclimate the skin through gradually increasing exposure.

The best protection from sunburn, especially in the unacclimated body is to use sunscreens. There are now many on the market. The key ingredient is para amino benzoic acid (PABA).

Fig. 4-3 Electromagnetic spectrum of radiation.

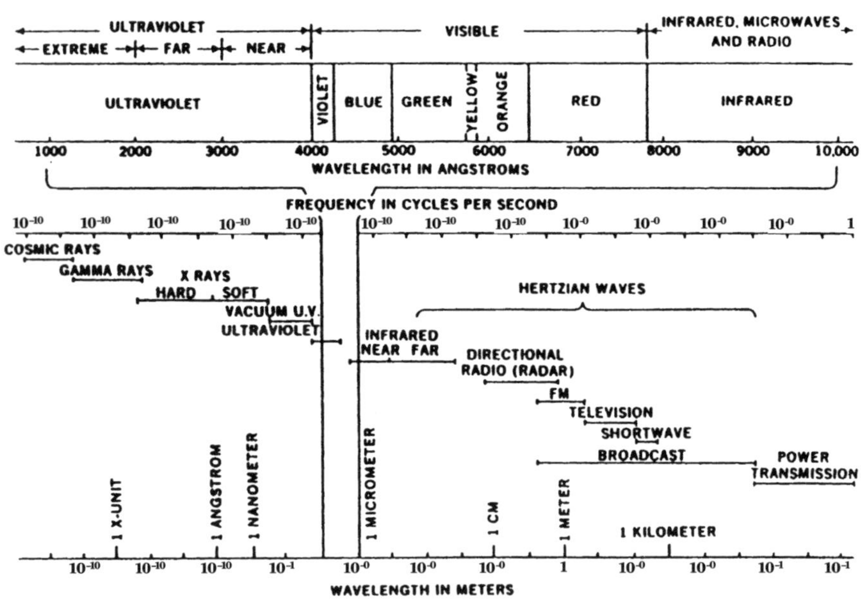

The more PABA in a sunscreen, the greater the level of protection. Some people's skin is more sensitive to the sun and requires greater protection. Obviously, this is not a problem if proper clothing is worn to protect the skin.

> *In studies being done at the FAA's Civil Aeromedical Institute, it has been determined that radiation does not represent a problem for aircrew at this time, no matter how much they fly. There is one exception, however. There are certain recommendations concerning occupational exposure that apply only to pregnant women. Female crewmembers flying long-haul missions (transglobal) need to be aware that they may be exposing the unborn child to radiation limits that exceed those recommended on a monthly basis. Studies are ongoing in this area of research.*

Self-Imposed Medical Problems 5

Tony had a cold so his doctor put him on medication and advised him not to fly. He called in sick for the trip, which meant his chief pilot had to fly. Two days later Tony's cold wasn't much better, but now the chief pilot had a cold, too, and the next trip would have to be canceled unless another pilot could be found. Tony wanted to make points with his boss, so he suddenly "got well," and told his chief pilot that he was over his cold and he would fly the trip for him. Tony's cold symptoms were still there, however, so he doubled up on his medication before he took off just to be sure he wouldn't be congested in flight. Two hours later, while making an approach to his destination, Tony was so lightheaded and unsteady (from the antihistamine medication) that the landing was too hard and he veered off the runway.

TEMPERATURE EXTREMES, illness, noise, weather, and several other situations that are beyond your control can affect your health and performance. There also are several circumstances over which you do have control, so any negative effects that they have on your performance may be unnecessary or self-imposed. How well you fly or function is compromised as a result of how you abuse your health or live your life. "Playing doctor," that is, making a self-diagnosis and then using self-medication is a common occurrence and made easier as a result of all the medications that are available to you in most every store. Also, overindulgence of alcohol, nicotine, caffeine, and other easily obtained abuses can easily impair your body's functions and your mind's ability to function safely. They are all self-imposed actions; nobody forced you to do them.

Playing Doctor

The primary reason that you see a doctor is because you are in pain, uncomfortable, or unable to work or play. You are looking for relief so you can go back to your activities. The doctor also wants you to feel better and has the added responsibility of finding out why you feel badly. More importantly, he or she must determine which conditions could be serious to your health and which ones could be ruled out as the source of your pain. Once this has been accomplished, the doctor can treat the cause, if it's treatable, and then, and only then, treat your symptoms. Unfortunately, the doctor is often bypassed because you don't want to take the time to see a doctor unless you are really sick. The following ailments are some of the more common ones for which you may be tempted to play doctor.

Colds and Flus

Colds and flus are commonly caused by viruses. Antibiotics do not cure viral infections as they do bacterial infections. Therefore, there is no cure for the cold or flu. Only time and allowing your body to fight off the viral infection ends the malady.

The symptoms of a cold or flu are what get your attention, and they can range from a simple sore throat and cough to generalized aches and pains, fatigue, headache, and congestion. Such symptoms, which are often limited to your respiratory system, are sometimes caused by bacteria and therefore respond to antibiotics. Therefore, if your symptoms don't begin to clear on their own in a few days, a doctor should be called so he or she can decide what the course of treatment should be, perhaps antibiotics.

Flus often have the same symptoms as colds, if the flu virus affects the respiratory system. Many flus, however, are associated with the gastrointestinal (GI) tract with resulting nausea, vomiting, diarrhea, and stomach cramps. Sometimes these symptoms include a generalized malaise (achy, tired, "feeling rotten"). These same symptoms, however, can result from problems with your gall bladder, appendix, liver, and other organs. Symptoms are not very good diagnostic tools.

For whatever reason, these are the symptoms that you often try to take care of yourself. Self-medication becomes easy because the marketing statements on the packages of over-the-counter (OTC) medications and drugs imply that they will clear up these symptoms and by inference, cure your problem.

If you feel that you aren't too sick, then it is very tempting to assume you're okay as long as you can take care of the symptoms with these OTC medications. But now you have three strikes against you—the effects of the cold or flu, the potential side effects of the medications (especially in flight), and the possibility that you made the wrong diagnosis.

Hayfever

Hayfever affects just about everybody to varying degrees, depending on geographic location and type of activities. Even though you may not consider that you have hayfever (or allergies), mild allergic-type symptoms are often mistakenly thought to be caused by a cold. The significant difference between the two is that a cold is an actual infection, even if caused by a virus, and this infection results in additional symptoms, such as fatigue and compromised performance skills, that are potentially unsafe in flight. Allergies may have similar symptoms, such as sniffles, sneezing, and even a cough, but it's uncommon to feel malaise.

Injuries

Because of your eagerness to fly, some injuries that are not considered serious to performance (e.g., minor broken bones, cuts, sprains, etc.) are often minimized. Arthritis and tendonitis, although not injuries, are experienced by just about everyone at one time or other, especially as they get older. Self-diagnosis of arthritis is common. Persistent symptoms from any of these conditions, however, are often an indication that there is more going on and a doctor should be informed.

A variety of OTC medications are available to treat the symptoms of these and other conditions, and to control the discomfort. Keep in mind, however, that medications are often used with the thought that in time the cause of the problem will go away anyway. Therefore, you rationalize that, by relieving the discomfort, you can return to flying. Furthermore, taking away the symptoms may mask the only signal your body has to alert you to a continuing problem.

There is a conflict, therefore, between your desire to fly and your willingness to accept that you may not be safe as a result of your medical disorder, whatever it may be. A simple statement from a doctor saying that your medical condition shouldn't interfere with flying may be misleading because many doctors are not familiar with the unique requirements and conditions for flying. That statement from a well-meaning doctor may give you a false sense of safety when, in fact, you are not safe. For example, a sprained ankle after several weeks is still weak but you do not realize that until you try pushing a rudder pedal in a crosswind landing.

There is also the philosophy that because others have tolerated the illness, used self-medication, and flown without apparent difficulty, it's okay for you to fly with the same illness. This reinforces the rationalization that you are safe to fly. Looking at the labels on OTC medications complicates the situation because of their claims to making your symptoms go away—the quick fix. The eagerness to fly the trip now overrides the potential of being unsafe during the flight.

A rule of thumb is that if you have any medical condition or symptoms for which you feel you need treatment, including OTC medications, then you probably aren't safe and you should reconsider flying. Ground yourself for a few days. Mild symptoms from known causes may be the exception, but only if you are sure of your diagnosis and an acceptable safe treatment.

Self-Medication

There is a huge market for medications and drugs that the public can purchase without a prescription or without visiting a doctor because of the perception of the "quick fix." Over-the-counter medications are a multibillion dollar business in the United States alone. Although the Food and Drug Administration (FDA) is charged with protecting the public from medications and chemicals whose labels mislead or imply false results, there is a continuous struggle to keep ahead of the false or misleading claims with factual information. Current programs of enforcement by the FDA to ensure legitimate labeling that is not misleading helps the buyer, providing the buyer reads the label.

Pilots and flight attendants are no exception to being vulnerable to the hype of the many ads for quick-fix medications. Although not deliberately seeking unsafe or unhealthy therapy, you are often swayed into judging that you know how ill you are and that you can fly safely. Thus, you self-diagnose and then self-medicate. Would you take a sleeping pill to cure a cold? You are when you use OTC medications.

Military flight surgeons and aviation medical examiners (AMEs) are often asked if it is okay to take a certain medication and still fly. The initial response technically has to be "No." There is no list of approved drugs or medications that you can use, prescription or OTC, without approval by a flight surgeon or AME. Obviously, there is a place for many medications and treatments, even OTC, but they must be taken only with the full knowledge of both you and your doctor as to why they are needed and their effects on safety and performance. It's a situation of risk assessment. Because civilian aviation doctors do not have a close relationship to the flight crew (like within the military), you must assume responsibility for determining what course of action to follow if you are feeling "under the weather." That's stated in FAR 61.53, which says that you must not have any disqualifying (unsafe) medical problems to be legal to fly. Thus, you must be healthy enough so that if you had to pass an FAA medical before you flew, you would meet the standards. Instead of playing doctor and if in doubt, check with your AME.

Marketing Claims

Reading the labels on the containers of OTC medications is often very revealing; they are sometimes creative in what is claimed. It's uncommon to find any comment about cure or coping with the *cause* of the symptoms. And, of course, there is the ultimate disclaimer that warns you to see your doctor if symptoms persist.

Consider some of these claims for OTC drugs:

- Symptomatic relief! Some symptoms are relieved but sometimes at the expense of causing significant side effects, especially in a flight environment. Symptom relief is an effective statement because that is precisely what you are looking for in the medication.

- Temporary relief! Temporary relief could mean a few minutes to a few hours. It does not mean permanent relief as is expected if the medication is curative.
- Extra Added Ingredients! This implies greater potency or more reliability in meeting its claims, even though that extra ingredient could simply be caffeine! The FDA is cracking down on claims that these added ingredients really do or do not do what is claimed. The label tells you only the names of the added ingredients.
- New and Improved! Compared with what? The ingredients probably are the same, but the amounts may be slightly different, or perhaps the only difference is the shape of the pill or the color of the liquid. It doesn't mean the drug is any more effective than the previous drug.

It would be a good exercise to go into a store, pick out a few common remedies, and read their labels just to see how creative marketing people can be to get you to buy their product.

Basic Ingredients

There are over 450 different drugs and OTC medications made from a combination of one or more of the chemicals noted in Fig. 5-1. These eight ingredients make up a high percentage of all of the usable chemicals that are allowed in OTC drugs. There are others, of course, but these are certainly the most common. In addition to discussing the effects and side effects, the label gives the half-life for each chemical. Half-life is that amount of time that half of the chemical needs to get out of your body leaving the other half. For example, if you ingest 1 gram of a drug and its half-life is 10 hours, then in 10 hours 0.5 gram would still be in your body.

Antihistamines

These chemicals are the most popular ingredients in OTC medications for allergies or colds. There are many kinds of antihistamines and several can only be obtained by prescription. Some of the more common antihistamines are brompheniramine, chlorpheniramine, doxylamine, and diphenhydramine. Note that each generic name ends in *-ine*.

Effects: Primarily, antihistamines help dry up secretions from upper respiratory mucous membranes (nose and sinuses) that cause the sniffles and postnasal drip (often also leading to a

Fig. 5-1 Ingredients contained in a majority of over-the-counter medications.

Chemical name	Half-life*	Actions and side effects
Caffeine	Varies	Stimulant (adrenalin-like) Diuretic (urine loss) Fatiguing Withdrawal anxiety
Aspirin	20 minutes	Analgesic (pain killer) Antipyretic (fever) Anti-inflammatory Tinnitus (ringing ears) Gastritis
Acetaminophen	3 hours	Analgesic Antipyretic
Dextromethorphan	Varies	Antitussive (cough)
Ephedrine and Phenylphrine	3 hours	Decongestant Stimulant (like caffeine)
Chlorpheniramine	6 hours	Antihistamine (allergy) Sedative Drying agent (secretions) Vertigo Blurred vision Increased heart rate Decreased coordination
Phenylpropanolamine	6 hours	Decongestant Stimulant Anorectic (appetite) Amphetamine-like Increased blood sugar Increased blood pressure

*It takes about five times the half-life to clear the body.

mild cough). In addition, some of the associated itchy nose and eyes and sneezing is controlled; however, antihistamines are usually effective only with allergies, not infections. There is still some dispute as to whether or not antihistamines actually help to alleviate cold symptoms.

Side Effects: Drowsiness and sedation are, by far, the most serious problems with any OTC medication that contains antihistamines. There are many accidents, incidents, and stories of pilots who were incapacitated in some way as a direct result of taking such medication. There are some prescribed antihistamines that, according to studies, do not cause drowsiness. The FAA certifies these prescription medications. If such treatment is necessary to keep you flying comfortably and safe, then the doctor must be a part of treatment and monitoring. And the AME needs to give you an okay to remain on medication.

Antihistamines' Recognized Side Effects
(in susceptible individuals)

Chills	Confusion
Irritability	Delusions
Headaches	Hysteria
Muscle twitching	Paralysis
Rapid heart rate	Neuritis
Tremor	Tinnitus
Insomnia	Blurred vision
Hypertension	Dilated pupils
Euphoria	Vertigo
Delirium	Double vision
Drowsiness	Heartburn
Fatigue	Nausea
Weakness	Constipation
Anorexia	Nightmares
Impaired judgment	EKG changes
Hypertension	Hypotension
Nasal stuffiness	Dermatitis
Dry mouth	Anemia
Hypoglycemia	Sugar in urine

There are many other side effects of OTC antihistamines that are unacceptable in flight. These include decreased coordination, reduced visual accommodation, dizziness, depression, and some cardiovascular effects (e.g., rapid heart rate, reduced vascular shunting response). In general, the use of any OTC antihistamines should be cause for you to temporarily ground yourself.

Sleeping Medications

It is important to note that virtually all OTC sleep medications are antihistamines! Drug companies have simply changed the name of the product, put a different label on the bottle or box, and the antihistamine now becomes a sleeping pill, exploiting its side effect of sedation. Would you take a sleeping medication to treat your cold so you could fly? That's what you would be doing.

Decongestants

Generally, decongestants are better tolerated than antihistamines. They are found in OTC medications, separately and in combination with antihistamines, and other chemicals. They are often the active ingredients in most nose sprays. Common decongestant chemicals are phenylphrine, ephedrine, and pseudo-ephedrine.

Effects: Mucous membranes usually swell during colds, flus, and allergies. This swelling causes congestion and plugging (blocks) in the nose, eustachian tube, and sinuses. Congestion is what creates problems in flight, often in the form of ear and sinus blocks. Decongestants may reduce this swelling. They do little to reduce secretions.

Side Effects: The major problem with decongestants is their stimulant effects, which are similar to those of caffeine. They include making you nervous, jittery, and overactive, plus keeping you awake when you are trying to get needed sleep. Most people are tolerant of these effects but it is difficult to predict what happens to an individual in flight. An already heavy load of coffee, plus the symptoms for which you need a decongestant, may increase impairment. Furthermore, pilots who have borderline high blood pressure should be aware that decongestants aggravate blood pressure elevation. It is wise (and expected of you) to confirm the use of decongestants with your flight surgeon or AME if you have blood pressure problems.

Nose Sprays

Nose sprays help reduce the congestion of the mucous membranes of your nose. Frequent use of short-acting (less than 3 hours) nose-spray decongestants can lead to what is called rebound. The spray itself can be an irritant to the mucous membranes of your nose. Thus, as the expected favorable decongestant action begins to diminish in a few hours, you take another "shot" of the nose spray to keep your nose clear. Over a period of a few days, the irritation caused by frequent use produces its own swelling and congestion. This is rebound. Longer-acting sprays (over 8 hours, as with oxymetazoline) may be better tolerated, especially if used for no more than a few days.

Some doctors may recommend that you keep a long-acting nose spray in your flight bag as a "get-me-down" treatment, when you get caught in flight with an ear or sinus block. This is not a recommendation to use the nose spray prior to flight because of a known cold or allergy because, as stated, if you think you need treatment before flying then you should not be flying. Keeping a nose spray available during flight for emergency use probably outweighs the risk of imprudent use. If there is doubt, don't fly or contact your AME.

Analgesics (Pain Relievers)

Analgesics are sold alone for the reduction of pain or in combination with other cold and flu medications. Discomfort (whether pain, aches, or malaise) generally is why you seek help from an analgesic, but these symptoms also could be nature's way of telling you something is wrong and that it isn't safe to fly. Therefore, it is important with analgesics that you consider why you need the medication. Unless you know for sure why you hurt, you need to discuss your problem with your doctor.

Aspirin: Aspirin is one of the most common of pain relievers, but it is a medication that has several other effects. It is an antipyretic or fever reducer, and an anti-inflammatory medication frequently used for arthritis and other inflammation problems. It is relatively safe if used as directed, usually with food or an antacid, and if you do not take more than the recommended dosage. Avoid taking any medications containing aspirin if you have any history of previous stomach distress or gastritis.

Acetaminophen: Acetaminophen is often the ingredient that competes with aspirin in the marketing OTC medications. It is also an effective pain reliever for some people and found in combination with other chemicals in cold and flu medications. It is not an effective anti-inflammatory treatment. It appears to be tolerated better than aspirin in people who have problems with gastritis.

Ibuprofen: Ibuprofen was once only a prescription medication but is now available as an OTC medication with a smaller dose in each pill. The prescribed medication is usually used for inflammation, whereas the OTC pills are for pain (the analgesic properties were found as a side effect when it was used for its prescribed purposes). This chemical is relatively well tolerated in most people, but a few people do notice side effects such as stomach distress and even ulcers, just as with aspirin.

Cough Suppressants (Antitussive)

In most cases, the active ingredient in cough suppressants is dextromethorphan, a fairly innocuous chemical that can assist in relieving coughs in some people. It has few, if any, significant side effects. Dextromethorphan is not the only ingredient used in cough medicines; derivatives of codeine are sometimes found in prescribed cough medication. Codeine, used in this formula, is a very effective antitussive agent; however, it is considered a narcotic, is mood altering, can cause drowsiness, and therefore is contraindicated in flying. Codeine also shows up in drug testing programs.

Extra Added Ingredients

Extra added ingredients include a variety of chemicals that may or may not enhance the other ingredients and their effectiveness in a product. The FDA is watching closely to determine if these additions truly do any good as advertised. Caffeine is one of the most popular added ingredients and is commonly found in combination with aspirin and in diet pills. Another is an antacid that basically helps overcome some anticipated side effects such as stomach distress. Alcohol is another common example, although not mentioned as an *active* ingredient. Alcohol is often used as a solvent for all the other ingredients. Up to 25% or more of some OTC medication is alcohol—that's a 50 proof drink.

Phenylpropanolamine (PPA)

Phenylpropanolamine is becoming well known in the pharmaceutical industry as causing some very undesirable effects. It's a common ingredient in a variety of OTC medications, such as diet pills, cold and flu relief, and allergy control. It acts as an antihistamine, a decongestant, and an anorectic (appetite suppressant). Depending on how it is packaged, it can do one or all of these functions. Phenylpropanolamine is also a very strong stimulant for some people, giving them a high similar to that of amphetamines. It can have a severe effect on blood pressure, often elevating normal blood pressure to the point where the diagnosis of hypertension is made. Drugs with PPA can interfere with sleep, cause headaches, dizziness, rapid heart rate, mood changes, and nausea. The FDA is taking special interest in this chemical because of its many adverse side effects. Even without the FDA's recommendations, this chemical is not safe to take prior to or during a flight.

Stomach Acid Reducers

For several years, your doctor has prescribed a variety of medications to control the formation of acid in the stomach, primarily for the treatment and prevention of active and recurrent ulcers. Now, the same medication is in OTC drugs for the treatment of hyperacidity or heartburn. Although this OTC medicine is well tolerated with few side effects when taken at the correct dosage, stomach acid reducers could mask the symptoms that are your first clues for the presence of an ulcer. As described in Chapter 12, the presence of an ulcer is disqualifying until proven to be healed. If you have persistent heartburn and require frequent use of an antacid or other stomach acid reducer, it's best to check with your doctor to be sure you don't have an ulcer. It's the same as taking an analgesic for chest pain that could be the first subtle sign of a heart attack.

There are some concerns that bear repeating when discussing OTC medication or self-diagnosis. The most important is, "Read the label." You will find the above-mentioned chemicals and ingredients in just about all of the common drugs used for symptom relief. You will notice that they are in varying doses and often associated with different symptoms. This description may be in small print. Because the scientific names of most of the chemicals of concern end in *-ine*, you can have a better idea of what you can expect in terms of helping or hindering your health. The bottom line is if the symptoms that you diagnosis as being a result of a cold, flu, or something for which you feel it is necessary to be treated with OTC medication, you probably are not safe to fly. If in doubt, check with your AME.

Caffeine

No matter where you find it caffeine is a drug that can have adverse effects on your body. It also ends in *-ine*, which indicates it could affect your performance as a pilot. In some people it's use becomes a mild addiction or, at the very least, a strong habit. Caffeine, like alcohol, when used to excess in some people, can cause a variety of physical and mental dysfunctions or impairments. It is one of the most common drugs that can be easily purchased over the counter as part of a variety of beverages.

Caffeine increases heart rate and rhythm, affects coronary circulation, constricts blood vessel diameters, increases urine production and excretion, and disrupts normal mental processes. It's most significant effects are stimulatory, and as such, it can interfere with sleep. Caffeine tolerance varies from individual to individual, some noticing few if any side effects, whereas others notice significant, undesirable symptoms, even with only one cup of coffee, and at unpredictable times.

Sources

The main source of caffeine is coffee and tea (Fig. 5-2). Regular brewed coffee has an average of 100 milligrams of caffeine per

Fig. 5-2 Caffeine content of various beverages.

Substance	Amount (mg)
Coffee, 5- to 8-oz. cup	
Decaffeinated, instant	2
Decaffeinated, brewed	2–5
Instant	40–110
Percolated	65–125
Drip	110–150
Tea, 5- to 8-oz. cup	
Bag, brewed for 5 minutes	20–75
Bag, brewed for 1 minute	15–50
Loose, black, 5-minute brew	20–65
Loose, green, 5-minute brew	15–60
Iced, canned	25–35
Cola drinks, 12-oz. glass	
Pepsi-Cola	38
Coca-Cola	33
Tab	32
RC Cola	30
Diet RC	25
Diet-Rite	17
Other soft drinks	
Mountain Dew	54
Dr. Pepper	38
Cocoa, 8-oz. cup	50
Milk chocolate, 1 oz.	3–6
Bittersweet chocolate, 1 oz.	25–35

cup. Decaffeinated coffee has only about 4 milligrams. Tea is another source of caffeine, with about 70 milligrams per cup (or glass of ice tea). Other caffeine sources include a cup of cocoa (50 milligrams), cola drinks (40 to 70 milligrams per 12 ounces), and chocolate (15 milligrams). Caffeine, as previously mentioned, is also present in many OTC medications.

Occasional caffeine intake in excess of 250 milligrams often is symptomatic in many people who have not built up a tolerance over the years. Symptoms become more noticeable in very sensitive people. Some pilots are not aware that some of their fatigue, headaches, and nervousness could be secondary to their caffeine intake, often when withdrawing from caffeine intake. Others notice a change in their heart rhythm, in addition to heart rate, with just one cup. This rhythm disturbance may show up on an FAA EKG. Because this rhythm change could be caused by something besides caffeine, a further evaluation could be required by the FAA.

Coffee is a strong stimulant, which, of course, is the reason most people use coffee, along with its taste. One to two cups per day is usually well tolerated and does, in some people, diminish fatigue, improve your mood and alertness, and temporarily increase mental and physical work capacity. The withdrawal effects, however, after a trip where a lot of coffee has been ingested, can be counterproductive especially in combination with the fatigue associated with the trip. Some experience withdrawal side effects from just 1 or 2 cups of coffee.

Side Effects

Because caffeine is a stimulant to the CNS, some people are unable to sleep even if they ingest caffeine several hours before retiring. This can be a real dilemma if you drink coffee to stay awake on a long trip and then subsequently try to get to sleep that night. For some people, only one cup of coffee or tea is enough to keep them awake if taken just a few hours before retiring.

Caffeine is a strong cardiac stimulant, acting like adrenaline to the heart muscle. Arrhythmias, such as skipped beats and other irregularities, may show up on a physical exam or an EKG, such as with a company or FAA exam. Pilots have been grounded for arrhythmias until the evaluation is completed satisfactorily and no other problems or causes are identified. To discover that your suspicious EKG was secondary only to your caffeine intake is more than just embarrassing. You probably already know how you respond to any caffeine. If the total is in excess of 400 to 500 milligrams per day, you can be sure you will eventually have some problems.

Caffeine is also a diuretic (increases urine production and excretion). Thus, one cup of coffee could result in urinating two or more cups of water. This could result in a negative fluid balance that makes dehydration even a bigger problem than usual. Remember that dehydration is a common occurrence in the cockpit. Because of an additional chemical called theophyline, a cup of tea can be a stronger diuretic than the same amount of coffee. Drinking ice tea, especially during the summer, may be refreshing but it also can be more dehydrating. Because of its diuretic effects in an already dehydrating environment, even before you go flying, you need a lot of water to rehydrate.

One of the most serious yet subtle side effects of caffeine is on mental functions, often called caffeinism. It can result in anxiety and panic disorders, headaches, nervousness, and worsens premenstrual syndrome (PMS). This becomes particularly true during withdrawal from caffeine. Swings of heavy intake (as on a trip or studying for exams or checkrides) to minimal amounts (during your daily routine when not flying) often generate problems not usually considered by you or your doctor to be associated with caffeine. Yet these symptoms must be considered abnormal until proven otherwise, which means yet another medical evaluation.

Tolerance

Low amounts of caffeine are generally well tolerated by most. Over a period of years, however, your body builds up a tolerance for greater levels. Although you may not be aware of symptoms of too much caffeine, your body is still reacting to those high levels and expects this added boost every day. If you are drinking more than three cups of coffee (or ice tea or cola products) per day then you can assume you could be at toxic levels, especially in the environment of flight where you are usually drinking more, even before and after the trip.

A good policy to follow is to have one cup of regular coffee in the morning but then either dilute subsequent cups or substitute decaffeinated coffee or tea. Actively increase your water intake, especially during flight. Suck on one of those large water bottles with the tube sticking out the top. Keep it in the cockpit. Substitute juices, herbal teas known to be safe, or just plain hot water (or hot lemonade, etc.).

Other Self-Imposed Problems

Hypoglycemia

Hypoglycemia is not a disease in the traditional sense; it is a condition of having low blood sugar for any number of reasons, often the result of the inability to find or unwillingness to take in adequate nutrition. Crew meals are often limited to calories from a vending machine. Restaurants, coffee shops, and fast-food places aren't always open when you need them, when you're in a hurry and don't have time (e.g., in the morning), or when the expected meal is not available on board the airplane. Missed meals are problematic and can have unpredictable results. Furthermore, you may not be able to control the unexpected lack of adequate and nutritious food. There are creative ways of "bagging" food, however, that you can keep in your flight bag or suitcase. Bagged food can range from a roll of candies to bags of peanuts or trail mix (peanuts, raisins, and candy) to easy-to-eat veggies. And don't forget your large glass of water. Such food is admittedly not as nutritious as a regular meal but it does resolve the symptoms of hypoglycemia for the short term and is certainly better than not eating at all.

By recognizing the symptoms of hypoglycemia, such as headache, stomachache, nervousness, or shakiness, then you can take appropriate corrective action. This includes some form of instant calories such as candy or the ever-present peanuts. Prevention is still the best therapy, respecting the need your body has for adequate calories that will last for several hours. Avoid consuming only empty-calorie food consisting mostly of sugar (e.g., sweet rolls and colas) to take the place of any meal.

The cola and candy bar, especially when substituted for breakfast, can often lead to a blood sugar rebound effect (sugar high in the blood followed in a few hours by a sugar low (hypoglycemia). Try to find foods high in protein for snacking. Even a quick cheeseburger for breakfast is better than sugary foods. A cheeseburger provides energy over a longer period of time and should prevent hypoglycemia and the rebound effect. Don't worry about the long-term problems with high-fat foods. You're eating such foods only to get you through the day.

Smoking

Aside from the risks to your health as described in the chapter on health, smoking also puts carbon monoxide (CO) into your blood system and cells. As explained in Chapter 2, CO interferes with the transportation of O_2, leading to even higher levels of hypoxia. Smoking up to three cigarettes prior to flight increases your body's hypoxic symptoms as if you were 2,000 to 3,000 feet higher—at an increased physiological altitude. This becomes a significant factor with night vision and performance.

Smokeless tobacco or chewing tobacco is a major source of nicotine. Tobacco puts more nicotine into your body than does smoking. It greatly increases your risk for other serious medical problems. A wad of tobacco in your mouth generates a lot of saliva, which is why you must either swallow or spit it out (Fig. 5-3).

Fig. 5-3 Self-imposed stress.

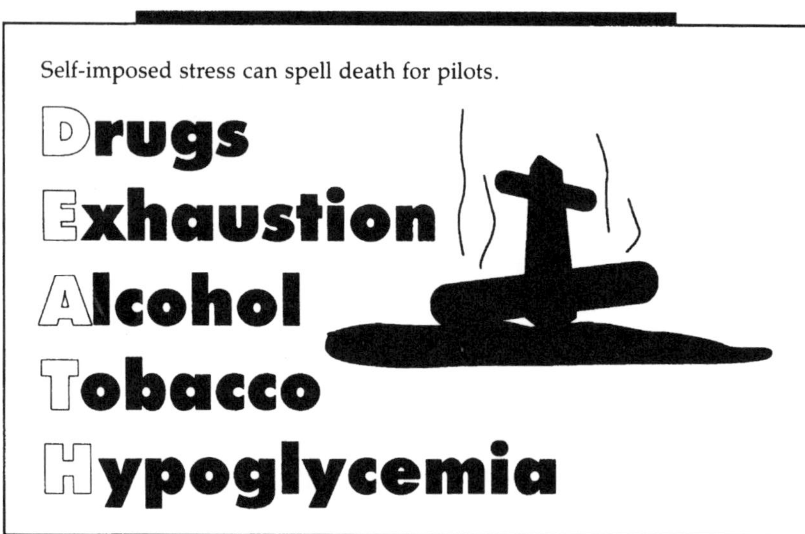
Self-imposed stress can spell death for pilots.
Drugs
Exhaustion
Alcohol
Tobacco
Hypoglycemia

Prescribed Medications

Although not self-imposed because your doctor feels you need to be on medication, it's important to know that there are situations when you can fly and still be on prescribed medications. Essentially, when deciding if you are safe, it is a combination of why you need the medication along with any side effects that would be present, just like with OTC medication. Remember, at altitude your symptoms may be different than at ground level. It is wise, therefore, to ground yourself for several days, determine if the medication is doing its job, and whether or not there are side effects. Sometimes unwanted effects disappear after several days on the medication. If the illness is under control and there are no significant side effects, then returning to flight status may be okay. Regardless, if the illness is significant enough to require medication, this situation must be coordinated with your treating physician and your AME or flight surgeon before flying.

Another problem is your schedule interfering with the timeliness in taking your medication. Or you just plain forget to bring your medications along on a trip. If you are supposed to take your pills four times a day, that doesn't mean one every hour for 4 hours in the morning before you take your trip. Your medication must be taken as directed on the container—it may not get into your system adequately if not taken as directed. Furthermore, it is important that you understand the required dosage and frequency of when you take the medication. Be sure to advise your personal physician about what your duties are in flight, let him or her know that you are a pilot, and then consider if flying is safe. It is essential that you fully understand the potential side effects, so you know what to look for and your doctor can advise you about your performance degradation. Once again, it there is any doubt, consult your flight doctor.

Alcohol

Before continuing with the topic of alcohol, it is essential that you have a clear understanding of FAR 91.17, which applies to all pilots. "Drugs" (as stated in the regulation) could include OTC and prescribed medications, in addition to the traditional definition of illicit drugs. Because "using any drug that affects" and "influence of" refers to alcohol and drugs, then this FAR takes on more significance for the pilot even after the legal 8 hours. It reads as follows:

A. *No person may act or attempt to act as a crewmember of a civil aircraft—*

1. Within 8 hours after the consumption of any alcoholic beverage
2. While under the influence of alcohol
3. While using any drug that affects the person's faculties in any way contrary to safety or
4. While having 0.04 percent by weight or more alcohol in the blood.

The remainder of this regulation refers to your passengers and to you submitting to testing for alcohol and drugs. Keep these regulations in mind as you consider whether or not you and your crewmate are truly fit to fly and legal.

DOT Alcohol Rules (5-15)

In addition to the FAA's rules and regulations relating to the use of alcohol, the Department of Transportation (DOT) mandates the following. Note that the consequences are more severe and that they pertain to all safety-sensitive work: pilots, flight attendants, dispatchers, and mechanics, to name a few.

PROHIBITED CONDUCT

- Pre-duty use within 8 hours of consuming alcohol from any source
- On-duty use is prohibited
- Reporting for or while on duty with alcohol concentration of 0.04 or higher
- Reporting for work with 0.02 to 0.039 must wait (not a violation)

CONSEQUENCES

- Immediate removal from duty

- Permanent disqualification from service for on-duty use, first event
- Permanent disqualification from service for pre-duty use, second event
- Report sent to Federal Air Surgeon
- Report sent to Airmen Certification Office

Alcohol and Other Abuses

Alcohol is found in a variety of items, including food additives, components of medications, and, of course, beverages. Alcohol is alcohol, no matter where it is found and it has the same effect on you whether it is in cocktails, beer, wine, or even punch. This may seem simplistic but there are many who feel that beer is only a beverage to quench thirst—like a soda—and they do not realize that several beers is the same as several cocktails as far as alcohol intake. There is a saying "If you drink a lot of beer, you drink a lot." Few summer beer drinkers would admit that they drink a lot of alcohol. The same holds true for wine. There is the same amount of alcohol in 12 ounces of beer, a 1.5-oz shot of vodka, or a 5-ounce glass of red wine.

Physiology

Ethanol (or ethyl alcohol) is the chemical name for the alcohol in beverages. It is readily absorbed in your stomach and small intestine. From there it immediately goes to your brain where most effects are noticed, some expected and desired, others unexpected and undesired. Other tissue cells become intoxicated with alcohol, sometimes replacing the water in the cell structure. Ninety-five percent of the ethanol is ultimately metabolized by your liver into CO_2 and water through a complex process. Prior to being broken down, alcohol is changed to glucose, a source of energy. Alcohol, therefore, is the ultimate empty calorie because it has no other elements of nutrition.

A full stomach often delays absorption but then alcohol lasts longer in your body. Liquors are absorbed quickly, whereas beer's alcohol takes longer to be absorbed. Carbonation, as well as sugar in the mix of a cocktail, increase the absorption rate. These variables make it difficult to determine how an individual responds to any given amount of alcohol. To say your body can tolerate greater amounts because some of these variations are controllable is naive. You have still ingested alcohol and your mental and physical tissues are still under the influence of or affected by the alcohol.

Alcohol in small amounts is excreted unchanged in the urine. Some is exhaled as a vapor from your lungs; this is a predictable amount and the basis for Breathalyzer testing. Therefore, the smell of alcohol on your breath is an indication that there is a significant amount of alcohol still in your circulatory system. This also means that there is still significant amounts in the blood reaching your brain and other cells. Even after your blood alcohol content (BAC) reaches zero, there is still impairment from the effects of a hangover and other physiological changes to be discussed later.

Basic Physiological Effects

Ethanol depresses the CNS and is probably the greatest threat of impairment to your performance. Fatigue and sedation are closely related resulting in a cumulative effect. Loss of inhibitions, increased euphoria, and a general sense of well-being are examples of how you feel and react with alcohol in your system. You talk more and at an increased volume and rate. You are more sociable, or at least perceive yourself as so. Performancewise, even at low levels of alcohol in your blood, there is a loss of your fine movement of muscles and touch discrimination—fine motor skills. There is also diminished memory and reduced concentration. Few people doubt that there is impairment. The unknown is to what degree there is impairment. There is increasing evidence that significant impairment exists for pilots even with a BAC of 0.02!

Ethanol is also a diuretic, especially in the early stages of drinking. As you approach intoxication, your kidneys tend to make less urine. The darker color of your urine is a good indicator of the amount of water that has already been lost through diuresis. The lighter the color of the urine, the more fluids you are currently losing. Eventually, your urine will be a deep yellow or orange, indicating that you are already dehydrated. This variation in the amount of fluids remaining in the body—the degree of dehydration—after the drinking is finished may have some effect on the severity of the subsequent hangover. Some studies indicate that fluid retention as well as blood vessel dilatation also causes the headaches and other symptoms that you experience the morning after.

Vasodilatation, or widening of the arteries, especially within the skin, is another effect. It makes you feel warm and gives some drinkers a ruddy or flushed complexion. As noted in Chapter 4 on heat and cold stresses, alcohol is counterproductive in coping with temperature extremes. By interfering with the body's attempts at shunting blood for controlling internal body temperatures, alcohol may make you feel warm, but you are actually losing heat.

Effects on the Body

Alcohol (ethanol) is a toxin to the body and to the liver, altering and killing tissue cells. Heavy drinkers lose about 100,000 brain cells per drinking day, which is about 10 times the normal attrition. We have billions of brain cells so in most cases, there is only minimal damage. The same is true with the liver. The cells are altered, ultimately turning into scar tissue. This is called *cirrhosis* and in severe cases is incompatible with a productive life, let alone normal metabolism. These changes to the liver (and also to the kidney) can be detected by changes in comprehensive blood test profiles. Thus, a change in liver function test results usually is considered secondary to alcohol abuse until proven otherwise.

An increased heart size, and elevated blood pressure and heart rate are some of the cardiovascular system's responses to excessive alcohol intake. Blood lipid levels (cholesterol, LDL, etc.) also are increased. A doctor seeing a patient with unexplained hypertension, rapid pulse, and elevated cholesterol often suspects alcohol abuse and suggests further testing. Irregular rhythms are common with intoxication and become chronic with heavy drinkers, even long after the last drink. This includes heart blocks, extra beats (PVCs—premature ventricular contractions), conduction defects, and tachycardia (rapid heart rate).

Alcohol is an irritant to the lining of your esophagus and stomach, sometimes resulting in gastritis. Gastritis is common with drinkers, who thus require large doses of antacids. At times the lining of the stomach develops an ulcer and sometimes they bleed. A medical emergency exists when you begin vomiting blood. It is very unpredictable when the stomach is going to be affected by your drinking. Once you have had an ulcer, you are at greater risk of developing a second one.

Ethanol also induces hypoglycemia long after the last drink. This effect, in combination with other nutritional shortcuts usually taken during the party and the morning after, makes you even more susceptible to the symptoms of hypoglycemia. Good nutrition with lots of water is the best way to help your body recover from alcohol poisoning.

Histotoxic hypoxia, where your body's cells are unable to use O_2, is often caused by alcohol. Within the cell, alcohol is a toxin, interfering with metabolism, especially with O_2. This is why your body acts as if it were at a higher altitude. Some have said that two drinks add between 4,000 and 8,000 feet to the physiological altitude in which your body is trying to perform.

Your vestibular system is also affected by alcohol, even for many hours after your BAC is zero. Your sense of balance and orientation is impaired. Dizziness is noted, especially during intoxication. When you lie down, the dizziness gets worse because the semicircular canals are tumbled. The latter effect includes a marked reduction in the tolerance to "G" forces (even mild) as experienced in a turn. Even with a BAC of zero, you can experience these impairments long after your last drink.

Effects on Performance

The most significant effect of alcohol intoxication is impairment of your fine motor or muscle skills and mental processes that are unique to flying. You are taught to fly straight and level but the greatest emphasis in your training is how to react in emergency situations. This often requires you to react instinctively while at the same time responding to rapidly changing situations. Rapid decisions and actions are necessary in a potentially deteriorating flight situation. Alcohol at even low blood levels interferes with every mental and physical activity associated with the skills necessary for a safe recovery.

Some of the impairments include increased reaction time, such as taking longer to make an evasive maneuver or correct an unsafe trim setting. Tracking is impaired, which equates into an inefficient and unproductive scanning of instruments. Judgment of distances and heights is compromised leading to inadequate situation awareness on approaches. Visual acuity is diminished, making charts difficult to interpret and closing traffic difficult to see. You may use incorrect settings on radios and navigation equipment. Coordination skills are seriously eroded, preventing you from doing several activities at once, as in a simple turn while adjusting throttle settings. You find yourself having to think about what to do next rather than acting instinctively, much like the effects of fatigue. Remember, these effects could still happen AFTER your BAC is zero!

The most subjective problem is your inability to think clearly and to make sound decisions. Like with hypoxia, you are unaware that your performance is impaired. As most pilots do, you are always monitoring yourself and seeking perfection. When that self-monitoring process is diminished by alcohol in your system, you are a prime target for unsafe situations. Alcohol allows you to do dumb things without even recognizing the seriousness of your actions or inactions. You take greater risks and your tolerance for unsafe conditions is widened.

When under the influence of alcohol, and you are a usually conscientious and careful pilot, you lose your normal attitude of caution when you see a change in your performance—especially in evasive maneuvers. Poor judgment is a by-product of this progressively dangerous situation.

All these impaired performance and judgment skills can be occurring at the same time and at a BAC of less than 0.04 percent, the legal FAA allowance. You may think you are doing better when in fact you aren't. And how are you going to tell? Even experienced pilots are impaired when faced with multiple tasks. And again, like being hypoxic, you are unable and unwilling to determine or recognize your impairment. Thus, you cannot and do not take corrective actions or let someone else fly.

Many more unsafe situations occur even when BAC returns to zero, and for many hours afterward. Couple this with the additional traditional effects of a hangover and you have increased your risk of becoming another accident or incident statistic.

Hangover

Hangover effects (post-alcohol impairment or PAI) are distinguished as separate from the direct and immediate effects of alcohol in your body just described. These symptoms include tremors, thirst, nausea and vomiting, heartburn, sweating, dizziness, and of course, headache. More subjective effects are increased irritability, anxiety, and mental depression.

With heavier drinking (without an established tolerance to large amounts of alcohol), these symptoms are more severe and mental function impairment is less subtle. Performance is affected in critical phases of takeoffs, landings, and emergency situations. There is marked reduction in your ability to perform nonroutine tasks. These impairments are noted even 14 to 24 hours after BAC is zero.

Hangover and Other Headaches
(Independent causes in *susceptible* individuals)

Hangover
- Excessive alcohol
- Red wine
- Cheap wine

Chinese Restaurant Syndrome
- Monosodium glutamate (MSG)
- Excessive salt

Hotdog Headache
- Sodium nitrite preservatives

Fermented Cheese and Salami

Dark Chocolate

Aspartame (NutraSweet/Equal)

Caffeine (withdrawal)

Consider: How often are two or more of these causes occurring at the same time?

A major problem even after BAC is zero is fatigue. Alcohol is known to reduce REM sleep (see Chapter 8), which means that you are not getting a restful sleep. You may be passed out or sleeping heavily but it is from depression of brain activity, not sleep. Obviously, the lack of sleep also causes fatigue.

Prevention of the effects of a hangover is related to decreasing the amounts and rate of ingestion of alcohol and reducing the absorption of alcohol into the GI tract. High-protein foods such as dairy products and meats stay in the stomach longer and slow absorption of alcohol. Gulping drinks increases not only the total amount of alcohol consumed in a given period of time but also allows the alcohol to enter the bloodstream and your brain more quickly. Carbonated beverages, including beer, tend to make your stomach absorb alcohol quicker. Thus, drinking juices and water instead of soda water is less likely to lead to a hangover. The slower the absorption, the slower the alcohol gets to the cellular level.

It should be obvious that 8 or even 12 hours "between bottle and throttle" is not nearly adequate to prevent the varied impairments from alcohol, especially considering the effects of a hangover. Impairment is dependent on the total amounts, the time over which alcohol is ingested, and the tolerance built up by you as a drinker. You could still be under the influence, as stated in the FAR, even if your BAC is zero.

The only cure for the effects of a hangover is the passage of time, sometimes up to 36 hours. Coffee and O_2 are not proven ways for reducing the PAI symptoms or for improving performance. Caffeine may make you subjectively feel better but may actually disrupt performance skills even more. Oxygen is not part of the metabolism of alcohol; however, the act of "sucking on O_2" may psychologically make you feel you are doing something to overcome the effects.

Tolerance of Alcohol

The body can develop, over time, a tolerance to very high levels of alcohol. Someone who brags that he or she can "drink you under the table" probably can but only because he or she has built up this tolerance. It is a significant indicator of someone who has a serious alcohol problem, no matter what the source.

Studies also indicate that you cannot tell by how you feel or perform when you are impaired or when your BAC is zero. In fact, as noted, some problems are unique even when alcohol is no longer present in your blood. Many pilots and flight attendants actually think they are safe to fly only 4 hours after their last drink, despite facts to the contrary. Often this is a perception based on their increased tolerance and the denial that they could be impaired.

Recognition of a Problem Drinker

It would seem easy to recognize a problem drinker by observing his or her drinking habits. It really isn't that difficult if you are honest with your observations. Few, however, want to be a snitch nor do they feel competent to pass judgment on someone they think has a problem, especially without clinical proof. After all, what is the definition of a problem drinker or one who is truly dependent on alcohol? Is it someone who drinks more than you? Or are there more distinct criteria? Anyone with a BAC of 0.15% is considered intoxicated but how often must a person be intoxicated before being considered an abuser or alcohol dependent?

The problem drinker has a little of all these indications. You must keep a high index of suspicion when you observe someone you know to be slowly developing a lifestyle that involves increasing drinking. Don't count on the flight surgeon or personal physician to intervene. It is estimated that less than 10 percent of referrals of alcoholics (or chemical dependents) to treatment comes from the doctor. Usually it's from concerned family and friends along with business and flying colleagues and managers.

Specialists in alcohol problems have specific guidelines to be used in determining if there is a potential dependency. The following are a few danger signals. In the right combination, these also could be diagnostic of alcoholism and cause for FAA medical disqualification.

A. EITHER OF THE FOLLOWING FACTORS

1. A clinical diagnosis of "alcoholism"
2. Evidence of withdrawal from alcohol

B. Any two of these major criteria that indicate that alcoholism is definite and a diagnosis of a history obligatory

1. A medical history of liver disease
2. A medical history of central or peripheral nervous system involvement
3. Psychological dependence on alcohol is demonstrated by either admission or by history
4. More than one conviction for an offense involving alcohol, including nonhighway arrests
5. Known to various health and social agencies in the community through contacts related to alcohol problems
6. Treatment at an inpatient facility devoted to alcohol rehabilitation

C. Minor criteria from which any three or four fulfilled or one major and two minor criteria

1. Accidents involving injury or property damage that may be presumed to be related to alcohol
2. Known to have a history of troubled relationships in employment
3. Known to have a history of troubled relationships within family
4. Known to have troubled relationships with banks or creditors
5. Intoxicated more than four times a year
6. At any time a BAC of greater than 0.2 percent
7. A history of blackouts
8. Odor of alcohol on the breath at the time of medical certification
9. Evidence of social and behavioral disruption

These criteria will be used as a guide to assist in determining the degree of use of and dependence on alcohol and whether or not there is a problem that could interfere with meeting FAA standards. Many of these criteria are also a sign of poor judgment in the use of alcohol. It would be difficult to convince anyone with some of these factors that they don't have a problem.

The two biggest indications for suspicion of alcohol dependency are increased tolerance to large amounts of alcohol and denial that there could be a problem. The denial is the hardest to define because the alcoholic is a master of denying that he or she can't control the drinking, even when confronted by other people with objective proof.

Addiction, dependence, and alcoholism mean somewhat the same thing for our purposes. The drinker cannot control intake, or is unable to say "enough." He or she is unable to stop after the first drink. Frequency of use is often daily with careful avoidance prior to work or flying. The amounts consumed are often staggering (literally); a quart of vodka or a case of beer per day are not uncommon. The deception to the drinker and those around him or her is the perception that he or she doesn't appear drunk or impaired. The drinker has developed a tolerance to large amounts alcohol without obvious outward signs.

Dependency is the main concern when discussing alcohol use, especially in aviation. The combination of being impaired (and not recognizing that fact) and the denial that there is a problem leads to the pilot or flight attendant often flying under the influence, even after BAC is zero. Therefore, identifying the problem drinker by keeping a high index of suspicion becomes the responsibility of everyone. Some things to look for include the following:

1. Increased tolerance to alcohol (probably the most important) resulting in drinking more and more rapidly than others.
2. Gulps the first drink or two.
3. A personality change over a period of time.
4. Increased absenteeism and use of sick time.
5. Increase in complaints about family life or management, often trivial and with a suspicious nature.
6. Frequently drinks alone and avoids nondrinking friends.
7. Increase in irritability, becomes more argumentative.
8. Denial of increased alcohol intake and of the problems just noted.

Treatment of Dependency

The first step in treatment is recognition, by both the pilot or the flight attendant and others. But the challenge remains—

few will take the step of recognizing that there is a problem and then taking action. This combination along with denial is often called *enabling*, allowing the problem to continue by enabling the drinker to continue through reasoning that someone else will intervene.

Once a problem is recognized and action is decided upon, the next step is intervention. Although it is hoped that the problem drinker will seek help, this is usually not the real-world scenario. An intervention is where concerned individuals participate in a structured intervention, an action that essentially corners the drinker into hearing what is happening to him or her, and what needs to be done. There is only one way out, only one solution for the drinker—to enter treatment, which must already be arranged. Intervention is often done by professionals, along with family and colleagues. More information relative to this step is best obtained from treatment centers, Alcohlics Anonymous (AA) representatives, and company employee assistance programs, etc.

Treatment for a dependent pilot must be at an FAA-accepted treatment center and usually as an inpatient (admitted into the center for the full term of treatment and not allowed to commute home). Treatment varies from center to center but generally follows the 12-step program developed by AA. Also, there is comprehensive testing, both medically and psychologically, counseling with professionals, and sessions with groups. The details can be obtained from the same resources just mentioned. It is recommended that you become familiar with the scenario to better appreciate how you can help. Even if you don't know an alcoholic now, chances are you will sometime in the future.

Alcohol, especially when associated with dependency is a major problem within all aviation. Often the only way aircrew members with a problem can be identified, treated, and returned to flight is through the combined efforts of those around them. The FAA will participate in this program if it sees the proper and appropriate efforts and results. Therefore, you are not ruining a pilot's career or flying status if the above-mentioned procedures are followed. There is no reason, in reality, to avoid intervention of a friend or family member. If you suspect he or she has a problem, seek advice from your company's employee assistance department, or union, or call the

FAA to obtain advice. (No names need be mentioned, you're seeking recommendations on whom to talk to, to get directions to help.)

Illicit Drugs

Illicit means *illegal*. Pure and simple. But for no other reason, if you are using these drugs, you are in violation of the law and federal regulations. It's not a matter of when they were used, how much was used, or how impaired you may have become. If caught you have no excuse. You broke the law. If you choose aviation as a career, illicit drugs are not acceptable nor are they tolerated.

That aside, there are some facts that you need to know, especially to recognize why these drugs are dangerous before and during flight. A prime problem with illicit drugs is their highly addictive properties. Furthermore, you can become more dependent on these chemicals than with alcohol, which means increased difficulty in achieving a successful treatment.

Kinds of Drugs

All these drugs are called mood-altering drugs and they are often considered stimulants, depressants, or hallucinogenics. Hence, there are families of drugs that are tested for in most drug programs: amphetamines, marijuana, cocaine, PCP, and opiates.

Marijuana is probably the most common of these drugs, although cocaine is equally common in some cultures and parts of the country. The active ingredient is delta 9 tetra hydrocannibinal (THC) and it is this chemical that is tested for in urine. The THC causes temporary euphoria and relaxation. More than with alcohol, it distorts perception, weakens critical judgment, and interferes with the ability to concentrate.

THC also increases heart rate and the incidence of cardiac arrhythmias. Short-term memory is impaired, IQ is thought to be diminished, and there is a decrease in reaction time and tracking (similar to effects of alcohol). In severe cases, there is marked depression and some hallucinations. Physiologically,

THC is stored in fat tissue; thus, it can be slowly released at unpredictable rates long after it is first taken into the body. The same effects can then develop with the greatest threat to the brain and this effect can occur up to 30 days after taking THC. Because most THC is taken in by smoking, THC smoke is far worse in producing cancer than regular smoking. THC also may cause genetic changes and damage and interfere with your body's immune system.

Testing

Using the current test reporting programs, there are no false positives for illicit drugs. The common procedure is a two-phased test for the five previously mentioned drugs (or their metabolites) in the urine. The first part is a screening test and it is here that false positives can occur. That is, some other chemical may show up as being positive for one of the five drugs. This positive, however, is not officially reported and a confirmatory test is automatically done by using gas chromatography and mass spectrography (GC/MS) analyses that generate specific curves for every known chemical. Therefore, if any one of the drugs is found to be present with this test, that drug is present because nothing else looks like that in the curves produced by the test.

Furthermore, it is necessary that the amount of the drug found must be at a level that must be surpassed. Thus, the test is not only qualitative but also quantitative. For example, if 90 units of THC were suspected in the screening test and the level to be considered positive is 100, then that part of the test is reported as negative. If above 100 units, then a confirmatory test is done. Again, there is a level above which that drug must be present before being reported as positive. That also means that there are drug users who won't be reported!

In conclusion, you have a lot more control of your health and how you perform in flight than you may recognize. Common sense, moderation, and recognition of self-imposed stresses can keep you out of trouble. Furthermore, you can assist others by advising them of the facts of self-imposed medical problems.

Vision 6

John, only 44 years old, had never worn glasses and he had passed his FAA exams without difficulty. He did notice, however, that it was more difficult to see the bottom line for near vision, but neither the nurse nor the doctor said anything about it. Because there was no limitation on his medical, John never thought he would have any problem reading for a long time yet to come. But tonight was different. He was tired from flying 9 hours across the Pacific as the copilot. The cruise was uneventful at FL390. The cockpit and instrument lights had been turned down because there wasn't much to do. Yet, he was having increasing difficulty reading the CRTs. The letters weren't clear and he had trouble telling 8s from 0s and 3s. Even reading the approach plate in anticipation of the arrival was less than sharp. Finally, he turned up the lights and there was an improvement. The captain noted the difficulty and offered his reading glasses to John. "Wow," he said, "does that make a difference! But I'm too young to be wearing these 'cheaters.' What's wrong?" All the captain said was to take a look at the cabin altitude and consider how long they had been flying under night conditions.

OF ALL THE SENSES used for flying, vision is by far the most important. In addition to supplying nearly 90 percent of your cues for orientation (vestibular and proprioceptive is about 10%), vision supplies data for monitoring your instruments, searching for traffic, and reading written materials, and it determines visual references for taxiing, takeoffs, and approaches to landing. Thus, any disruption of your vision virtually incapacitates you and impaired vision increases the likelihood of an unsafe flight. The effects of fatigue, hypoxia, minor illness, low light, dehydration, and other physiological decrements add to the loss of visual acuity. The other bottom line is lost situation awareness.

Most people take vision for granted, as long as they can read and see distant objects. But without testing for visual acuity, you have nothing by which to compare your vision and you may not be aware that what you are seeing is not as clear or sharp as possible. A common comment by children who begin wearing glasses for the first time is the realization that brick walls have lines. Until they began to wear corrective lenses, the bricks were blurred together and with nothing to compare this image to, it was assumed that there were no lines or separations between the bricks.

The same holds true for older pilots (usually over age 45) who begin to wear reading glasses for the first time. It's almost startling to them to see with such clarity their approach plates and CRT/LED characters. They may have been able to pass the FAA vision test but that didn't mean they were seeing near objects clearly. An interesting exercise in the doctor's office, after the initial eye exam, is to let an older pilot try reading glasses for the first time and then take the reading test over again. It makes him or her recognize what was being missed.

Furthermore, pilots with 20/20 day vision may not have adequate night vision as a result of the physiology of how the retina converts light energy into electrical energy for the brain. There also appears to be individual variation in pilots as to how light energy is perceived by the brain and translated into data necessary for flight. Thus, with the same visual acuity, one pilot sees better and uses vision more effectively than another.

Light and Lenses

Light, defined as radiant energy, excites cells of the retina of your eye. An electrical current is produced that is transmitted to the visual cortex of your brain for interpretation (Fig. 6-1). Visible light is only a small part of the radiation spectrum, ranging from the color of violet at 380 millimicrons (one millionth of a millimeter) to red, which is 760 millimicrons. Longer wavelengths (infrared) produce heat and are a source of increased energy. Damage to your eyes, especially the retina, is dependent on the degree of brightness and duration of these forms of energy.

Light rays (or energy) reach your eyes either directly from a light source or as reflected light from a source back to your

Fig. 6-1 The electromagnetic spectrum.

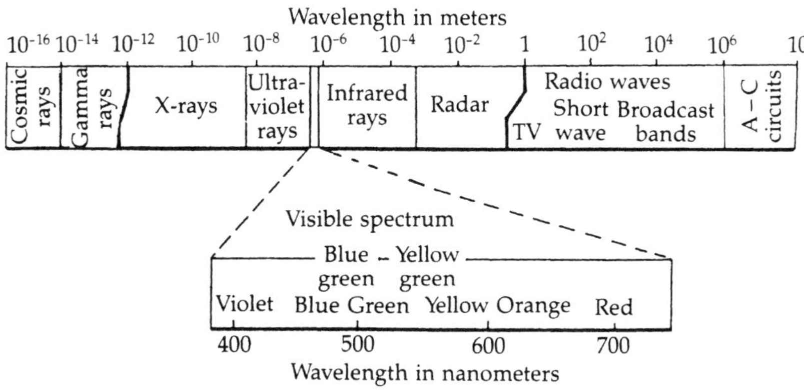

eyes (e.g., from water or snow or off a sheet of paper). There are individual light rays reaching your eyes from the light source (or reflected from an object). These rays are virtually parallel to each other beyond 20 feet from your eyes. Light rays originating closer than 20 feet come to your eyes at an angle.

Anatomy of the Eye

Light enters your eyes through the cornea, which refracts (bends) most of the light rays and then passes the rest into the lenses, which fine-tune the focus of the rays onto the retina (Fig. 6-2). The retina translates this radiant energy into electrical energy by photosensitive cells called *rods* and *cones*. Anatomically, your eyes are an extension of the brain and as such, the cells of the eye are adversely affected like any other brain cells by fatigue, hypoxia, and alcohol, etc.

The outer layer of cells of the eyeball is the cornea. The transparency of the cornea can become affected and permanently cloudy with age and with overexposure to ultraviolet radiation.

Like a camera lens, the lens refracts light rays as they enter your eye and focuses each ray onto the retina, which is analogous to the film in a camera. If the focal point (the point when

Fig. 6-2 Anatomically, the eye is an extension of the brain, so, like other brain cells, the cells of the eye are adversely affected by fatigue, hypoxia, and alcohol.

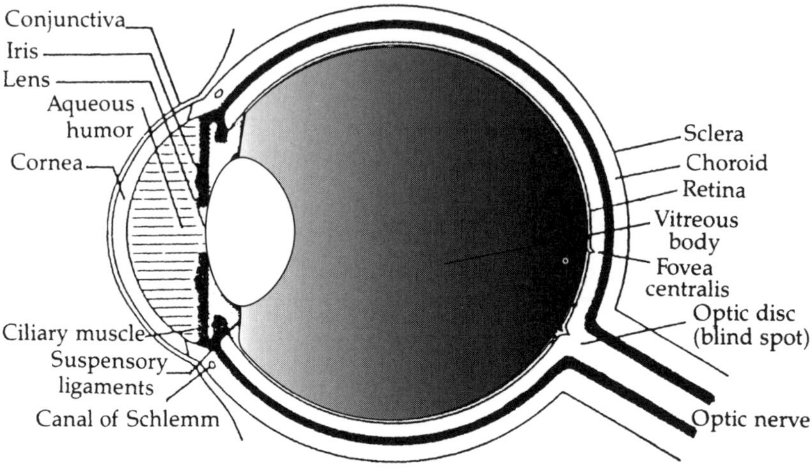

an object is focused) is in front or behind the retina, the perception is a blurred object. Because the lens of a camera is hard, a camera changes the focus by shortening or lengthening the distance of the lens from the film. The lens of your eye is soft and moldable and its shape is changed by the ciliary muscles that surround it. When these muscles contract or relax, the lens changes from fat to thin, allowing for more or less refraction of the light rays. Therefore, focusing is accomplished by changing the shape of the lens rather than changing the distance from lens to film. The distance in the eyeball is fixed. How well your lens can change shape determines how well your eye can clearly focus the visualized object onto the retina.

The lens can become opaque in some people as they age, resulting in cataracts. Also, as you age, your lens begins to stiffen and becomes less pliable, which prevents adequate changes in the lens shape and slows down the rapid change of focusing from distant to near objects (accommodation).

The iris is the colored membrane seen in the front of your eye, and it determines eye color. The center portion is called the pupil and, like a camera's aperture, the size of the pupil can be changed to allow more or less light to enter your eye. This gives your eye more flexibility to control the amount of light reaching the retina, wider in low light, smaller in bright light.

The brighter the light, the smaller the pupil, which, like a camera's aperture, increases the depth of field. Depth of field is the distance from the lens within which everything is in focus. Therefore, in low-light conditions, the depth of field is very small because the pupil is larger. Squinting duplicates this action to a small degree and allows for some focusing even without needed glasses.

The retina is the "film" of your eye; it uses photosensitive cells to detect light energy in place of light-sensitive silver nitrate crystals as in photographic film (Fig. 6-3). A unique difference is the distribution of two different kinds of cells within the retina. Each of these cells connects to a single nerve that in turn ends up in a bundle of nerves called the *optic nerve.*

One kind of cell is the *cone* cell, which is sensitive to bright light and colors and is involved in clarity. Cone cells are thus used primarily in the daytime and provide the most accurate visual sensing. Cone cells are highly concentrated in a small area called the *fovea,* the spot on the retina where most visual objects are focused, also called central vision.

Fig. 6-3 Anatomy of the eye.

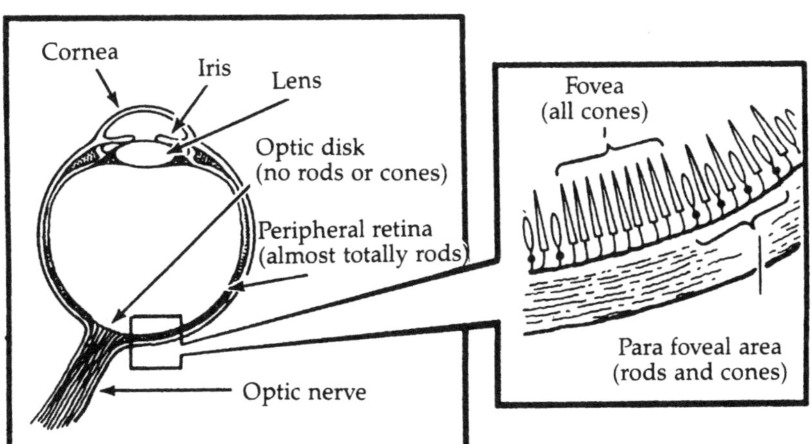

Rod cells are reactive to low light but not to colors; thus, they are more suitable for night vision. Surrounding the fovea is an increasing number of rods and a decreasing number of cones until at the periphery, there are no cones. This peripheral vision is more suited to orientation and is supplementary in night vision.

There are no cones or rods where the optic nerve is formed on the retina. This becomes a blind spot in vision but it is compensated for by having two eyes, each one overcoming the other's blind spot.

Optics and Physics of Light

A single light ray has a variety of physical properties that are associated with vision. Refraction is the property of a lens to bend the light ray so it reaches a given focal point (on the retina). Several light rays also must remain in focus through the same lens. Furthermore, the lens must be able to focus on a near object as well as on distant objects. This is called *accommodation,* wherein the refractive powers of the lens automatically change and allow for continuous focus as opposed to a camera that has to change the distance between lens and film.

Several other physical properties determine the clarity of

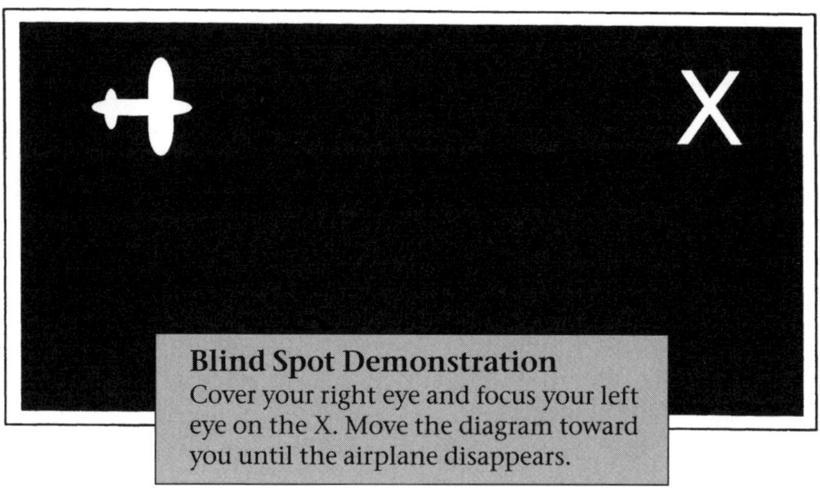

Blind Spot Demonstration
Cover your right eye and focus your left eye on the X. Move the diagram toward you until the airplane disappears.

the perception of these images even when focused. These include brightness, contrast, and color. Reaction time, or the time from seeing or identifying an object and recognition by the brain, also must be considered. In addition, atmospheric conditions such as fog, haze, and rain can interfere with light-ray clarity and transmission through the atmosphere. Such interference or diffusion of light rays results in illusions of erroneous distance and size.

The brighter the light either from a source or reflected from an object, the easier for your eyes to gather light rays onto the fovea. As with sound, low sources of energy results in a poor signal and with vision, lack of clarity or discrimination. The tradeoff is too much light and glare, which interferes with proper acuity and is also uncomfortable.

The greater the difference between an image of an object and its background (i.e., contrast), the easier it is to distinguish the object (or character). If the edge is fuzzy for any reason, the object appears out of focus. Look at a painting and you will notice how the artist has clarified (focused) the edges by outlining with a darker color. Fog and haze interfere with contrast and lead to poor acuity and clarity as well as to visual illusions.

Color also affects acuity. Each color is refracted differently through the lens as evidenced by the rainbow effect from a prism. Therefore, some colors, other than white light, which contains all colors, will not be focused relative to other colors. Red, for example, is refracted much less than other colors, which leads to an unfocused image, compared with an image illuminated by other colors or with white light. Therefore, using red light in the cockpit is not recommended because small characters on maps and checklists can be misread. They are not clear and sharply focused with other characters on backgrounds of different colors.

Two objects of the same brightness can be easily distinguished if there is a color contrast, even in low light. The clearest is black against white. Few situations, however, have such a clear definition. If you are not sure what is being visualized, you take more time than necessary to discern the nature of the object. Is the character a B, a 3, an 8, E, or 0?

Getting to 20/20

There are several variations of the lens that affect acuity. *Acuity* means the sharpness or keenness of vision—the ability to discriminate and recognize true shape and design—with perfect vision meaning that your eye sees or perceives exactly what the object is, whether it is close to or distant from your eye. Because focusing and accommodation are relative to the status of the curvature of the lens, you can supplement the curvature with artificial lenses (glasses or contacts). These focused light rays are signals to the brain for interpretation. Any loss of acuity results in a confusing interpretation of the significance of the object seen.

Variations of Acuity

Testing for acuity is accomplished by comparing what you can clearly see in actual conditions with what a normal eye with perfect vision can see in the same conditions. The eye doctor will have you distinguish various characters of different sizes. The bottom line of the eye chart (20/20 or 20/15, depending on the chart) can be read without difficulty by a normal eye. As the ability of your eye to see well diminishes, however, the characters must be larger, as in the second line (20/30). This means that the poorer eye can only see a character size that a normal eye could see at 30 feet. These tests are done under ideal conditions with bright light and black and white contrast.

Myopia is the most common acuity problem and is also called *nearsightedness* (Fig. 6-4). This means distant objects are out of focus without correction. Optically, the focal point of the lens is in front of the retina. When the point of focus is behind the retina, it is called *farsightedness*, and the near image is also out of focus.

Astigmatism is the unequal and variable curvature of the lens and the cornea that prevents an equal focus of varying distances. For example, a vertical light pole may be in focus but the horizontal power lines may be out of focus. If you have a perfect spherical cornea and lens, there is no astigmatism.

Fig. 6-4 Myopia (nearsightedness).

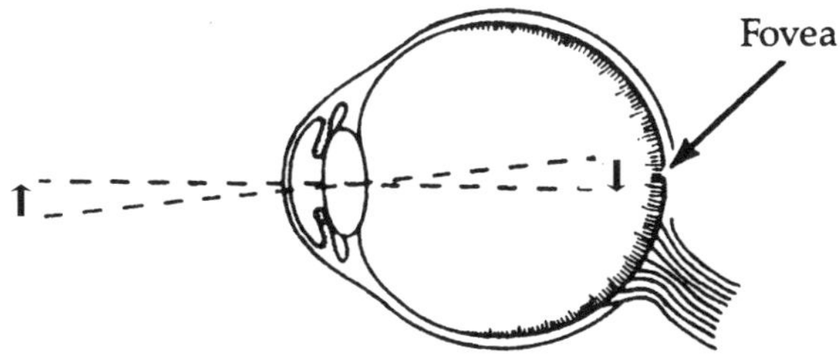

Presbyopia is a predictable change to your lens occurring as you get older. The lens stiffens and is unable to accommodate effectively (i.e., focus from distant to near). This condition affects near vision, which requires reading glasses for correction, whereas distant vision remains unchanged. There is also less light passing through the lens as you age, which further interferes with acuity. It is common for an older pilot to have uncorrected distance vision remain at 20/20 but need glasses to read. All pilots eventually need reading glasses.

Refractive Error

The refractive powers of the lens can be measured to determine how well it can focus by bending the light rays. This is accomplished by the eye doctor using a variety of different-strength supplemental lenses placed in front of your eye. You then tell the doctor which lens makes a character clearer on a chart that you are visualizing. Corrective lenses can be ground using this refractive error, such as +1.50 × –1.00 × 45, when stated as a prescription. The meaning of the numbers is unimportant in our discussion. this is just an example of a refractive error or glasses prescription.

Corrective Lenses

Once the refractive error is defined, lenses can be ground to correct for the error of refraction, allowing the focal point to be on the retina and in focus. This correction can be in the form of frame glasses or contact lenses. There are tradeoffs between the two. Frame glasses are generally more easily tolerated, whereas contact lenses allow for better peripheral vision. Also, as you get older and near vision changes, you may need to wear glasses for near acuity. If you already have distant vision glasses, then bifocals are needed.

Bifocal glasses (one part of the lens ground for distant and the other, lower part for near vision) are commonly worn but you need to get used to them. Furthermore, as it becomes more difficult to accommodate, even middle or intermediate distances may need correction; hence, trifocals. Your glasses may have to be specially ground to effectively accommodate to focal lengths not common outside the cockpit. This means that the control panel is usually farther away than for what most glasses are used. Many pilots are reluctant to wear glasses, especially for reading; however, the sooner such glasses are worn as a habit, the easier it is to adapt to the correction.

Some eye doctors prescribe monovision contacts, in which one contact is made to correct for distant vision in one eye and for near vision in the other eye. Over many hours, the brain starts to translate the two different inputs as one. These lenses, however, are not acceptable to the FAA, primarily because of the adaptation time necessary between using and not using these contacts. In fact, the use of such a combination was causative in an airline accident in 1997.

Night Vision

Vision under low light is a different physiological activity than under bright light. There is a chemical change within the cells of the retina that process light energy. During the day and in well-lighted conditions, most light rays are focused on the fovea, which is concentrated with cone cells and some rods. These cells have a chemical called *iodopsin* that allows the eye to be immediately stimulated.

Another chemical, *rhodopsin* or *visual purple*, is found in the rods. Rhodopsin must be made by these cells whenever light levels are low. Time is required for rhodopsin to be formed, which means it takes longer (up to 45 minutes) to adapt to low light than to bright light (about 10 seconds). Therefore, the retina has the ability to adapt to different light conditions by changing the amount of low-light-sensitive chemicals found in the rods.

Types of Vision

Because of the resources that the eye and retina have to adapt to in changing light conditions, your vision is divided into two types, depending on the amount of light available.

Photopic Vision

Photopic vision is used under daylight conditions with relatively sufficient light to activate your foveal cells (cones), either from sunlight or from artificial illumination. Color is easily discerned and images are sharp because of the fovea (central vision). Both rods and cones are found in the fovea but visual purple is bleached out by the light. Thus, photopic vision primarily uses cones and central vision.

Scotopic Vision

Scotopic vision occurs in low-light conditions, either at night or in darkened environments. Cone cells are ineffective, resulting in poor resolution of detail. Visual acuity decreases considerably, sometimes as much as 20/200. Color vision is totally lost.

Dark Adaptation

Dark adaptation is the process by which your retinas increase their sensitivity to decreasing levels of available light. Changes in visual purple or rhodopsin occur in the rods as the cones become less effective. The lower the starting level of available light, the more rapidly adaptation occurs.

It takes about 30 to 45 minutes for this adaptation in minimal light conditions. The lower the surrounding light, the longer it takes to adapt. Dark adaptation is also dependent on ideal conditions during which there is no exposure to bright light, even for brief periods. This bleaches the visual purple in the rods, which then have to be re-adapted. A very bright light, such as from a flashlight shone directly into the eye for even a second or from strobe lights on aircraft, can seriously impair night vision. Recovery could take several minutes.

Preserving Night Vision

The obvious technique to preserve night vision is to avoid bright lights and stay in a darkened environment for the time it takes for the rod cells to adapt. There is another method to protect your night vision and that is by using red light for illumination.

Rod cells in the retina are least affected by the light wavelength in the red range (long wavelengths). This means that a red light source does not bleach the rhodopsin as do other colors of shorter wavelength. It follows that the use of red light, once vision is adapted to night, would not alter the status of the retina and the rods. Thus, wearing red goggles in certain situations prior to actual flight and in preparation for a trip at night may be helpful.

There is a tradeoff, however. Red light refracts less than white light (remember that white light is a combination of all colors). Objects are no longer in focus by using only red light and it is more difficult to accommodate from near to distant vision. Red light also masks any red-colored objects, instruments, or map markings. As more and more CRT and LED displays are used in glass cockpits with multicolored and multihued characters, red light (or any light source other then white) becomes counterproductive and should not be used.

A good compromise would be to use red light only when trying to enhance the adaptation process, but not during actual flight. Low-level white light on the instruments and within the cockpit is the best, provided the intensity can be controlled. As darkness outside increases and the eyes adapt more to low light, a white-light source can be reduced.

Techniques for Improving Night Vision

There are significant changes in how your eyes perceive any level of light as darkness increases. Central vision is compromised because of the dependence on cone cells. Your peripheral vision becomes the primary source of visual cues (Fig. 6-5). Therefore off-center vision must be used, which involves looking at an object about 10° away from the object. This allows your peripheral vision to be the source of light signals to your brain. Another challenge is the observation that if an object is visualized for more than 2 or 3 seconds, the retinal cells can become bleached and the object can no longer be seen. Continuous scanning or changing position of your eyes on an object can prevent this occurrence (Fig. 6-6).

Color vision becomes less dependable as darkness increases. Colored lights from beacons, runways, and wing tips are discernible if the light source is strong enough to activate the cone cells. Other colors outside (and often inside) a dimly lit cockpit, however, appear as gray.

Reaction time of visual accommodation, recognition, and action also is impaired. This time is defined as that necessary to first recognize that an object is present and obtain visual contact. Additional time is necessary for this signal to get to your brain cells, which deal with vision, and the time necessary for your eye and head to turn toward and focus on the unknown object. Your brain must determine the importance and signifi-

Fig. 6-5 The central area gives the most acute vision in light down to the intensity of moonlight. Below this level of illumination, central vision cannot function as well and the central area is nearly blind. Any object that an individual looks at directly is not seen clearly.

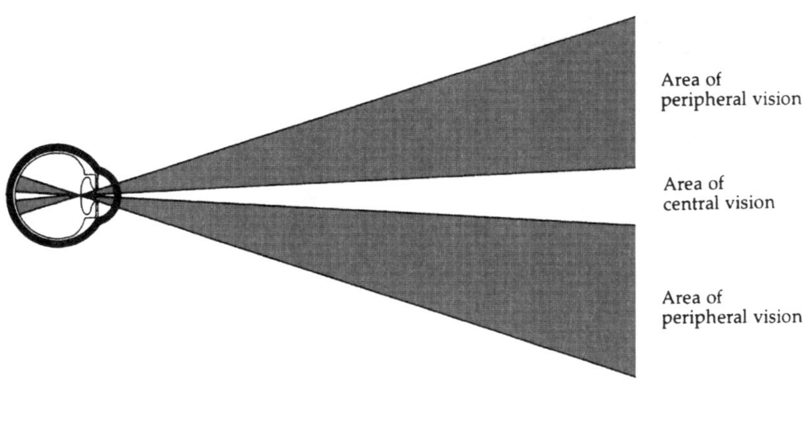

cance of the object's presence and further time is necessary for your body to react, such as by moving muscles to take corrective action at the controls. This whole process can take up to 2 seconds, depending on the conditions of the environment and your fitness. Exposure to extreme glare (e.g., from snow, sand, and water) during the day impairs dark adaptation.

Fig. 6-6 As darkness outside increases, off-center vision must be used.

Eccentric fixation

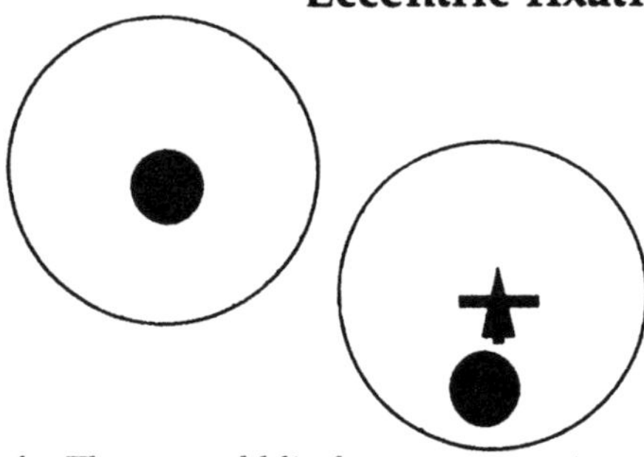

Left—The central blind spot present in very dim light makes it impossible to see the plane if it is looked at directly.
Right—The plane can be seen in the same amount of light by looking below (as is shown here), above, or to one side of it so that it is not obscured by the central blind area.

Dark adaptation

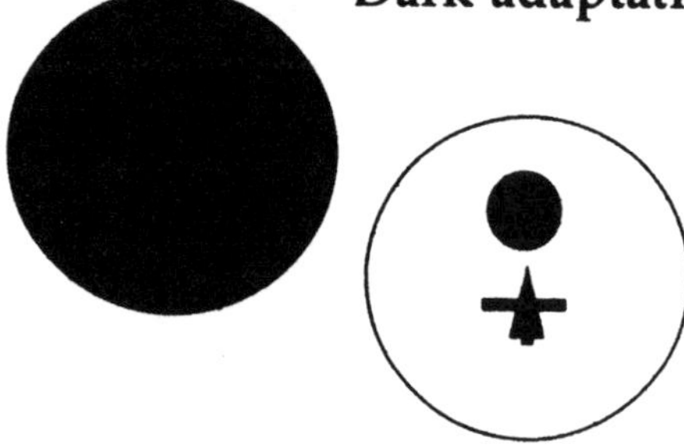

Left—View seen by a person who is not dark-adapted.
Right—The same view seen by a dark-adapted person who is looking at a point above the plane.

Seeing in the Bright Sunlight

Whether or not correction is needed for acuity, sunglasses are part of the image of the pilot. Sunglasses are often worn for cosmetic reasons only. As a result, there are several considerations that must be recognized when discussing the safe use of and the need for sunglasses.

The primary reason to use sunglasses is to reduce the amount of light from bright sources (the sun being the most obvious) to a level that is comfortable, yet doesn't affect the requirement for adequate visualization. Also, sunglasses reduce the glare that would impair adapting to nighttime flying. Additionally, there should be no distortion of color. This translates into ensuring that all wavelengths of light rays enter the eye for comprehensive interpretation. At the same time, sunglasses should filter out harmful ultraviolet and infrared radiation.

Because sunglasses decrease the amount of light entering your eye, the eye reacts by opening the iris (aperture) to allow more light onto your retina. Remembering the analogy to a camera, a larger opening or aperture decreases depth of field, which means that objects remain in focus but in a shorter depth. Professional tennis players rarely wear sunglasses because they do not want to compromise depth of field, which allows them to clearly see their opponent's tennis ball without having to rely on the focusing mechanism. This same principle holds true in aviation, especially in the traffic pattern.

Some of the specifications for sunglasses include maintaining a reasonable amount of filtering out light, probably no more than about 15 percent. About 85 percent of light transmission to the eye should be blocked. Wearing sunglasses in low light results in a definite loss of visual acuity from lack of adequate light energy. Some of the glasses that automatically darken in bright light should not be used in the cockpit because of the varying levels of light—from looking outside to reading instruments deep in the cockpit. Such glasses have a delay in the change (the lens could still be dark when looking in the cockpit) and they block less than 50 percent of light transmission, defeating the purpose for wearing sunglasses.

Sunglasses should be neutral in color, allowing most wavelengths to pass through. Any colors other than neutral gray could distort the image. With so many controls, CRT and LED characters, and maps in various colors, it is not safe to wear any glasses that filter out key colors.

A popular color for sunglasses is yellow or amber (blueblockers), which claim to make it easier to see through fog or haze. There is a perception of clearer visibility and sharper focus but this is more subjective than proven. Whatever the color of the lens, that color will be washed out when it reaches the eye. With vision a key source of sensory input, anything that is not a true color can mislead your perception of objects.

Polarizing glasses are also of dubious use in aviation. They are helpful in situations of high glare from reflected sources such as water, snow, and sand, but the tradeoff is distortion of light rays passing through the windshields, which are often plastic laminates, resulting in distortion of the images.

A final consideration is filtering out or absorbing UV and infrared light rays. This is easily accomplished by ensuring that the sunglasses state that they filter out UV light, especially the full range. The coating on these sunglasses is inexpensive.

Factors Affecting Visual Acuity

In either day or night flight, there are factors, many controllable, that can seriously affect the efficiency of your vision. This impairment is more noticeable during night flights than day flights. Hypoxia is the most important impairment because your retina is an actual anatomical extension of the brain; thus, anything that affects your brain immediately affects vision. Lack of O_2 affects brain tissue first. Thus, vision is concurrently eroded by reduction of sensitivity of rod cells. Low-light conditions add to this erosion. Hypoxia also increases the time necessary for dark adaptation. Such impairment is noticeable starting at about 5,000 feet AGL to which you are acclimated.

Carbon monoxide, which builds up in the blood in all smokers, creates hypoxia with the same results. Some have observed that smoking just three cigarettes adds enough CO to the blood cells to simulate an additional 5,000 to 8,000 feet of altitude to the body. Because alcohol can cause histotoxic hypoxia, the same reduction of acuity results even hours after the last drink.

Visual Illusions

From a purely visual perspective, many illusions are a result of distortion of light rays as they pass through air containing fog, dust, haze, etc. These components tend to refract or bend the light rays differently before they get to your eye, causing poorly focused objects, reduced light, and distorted visual cues. Visual cues often refer to objects of known size compared with unknown objects and they are especially noticeable in judging relative size and distance. Basic optics states that distant objects appear smaller than near objects. The distance of an object from a person is therefore a mental judgment com-

Visual Cues

Some of the standard monocular (one-eyed) depth cues an individual uses to judge distance are:

- **Linear perspective**—As objects get more distant, they appear smaller.
- **Aerial perspective**—As objects get more distant, they appear hazier.
- **Superposition**—Objects nearer to you obstruct the view of distant ones.
- **Brightness**—Nearer objects are usually brighter than distant ones.
- **Shadows**—With respect to the light source, nearer objects usually cast shorter shadows than distant ones.
- **Texture**—Nearer object appear "grainier" than distant ones; the level of detail increases in nearer objects.

paring size with already known comparisons or nearby known objects. Distortion of these light rays confuses your brain when trying to interpret size and distance. Furthermore, definition of edges is diminished, again resulting in poor discrimination of what you are visualizing.

Space Myopia

Space myopia is sometimes called *empty field myopia* and means that there are no objects on which to focus beyond 20 feet. Therefore, unless your eye and lens are stimulated into focusing, the lens tends to go into a resting state, focusing somewhere between near and far. As a result, outside targets are missed and the reaction time to accommodate to cockpit objects is somewhat impaired. Space myopia is easily avoided and corrected by frequently picking out an object beyond 20 feet such as a wing tip or a cloud edge and consciously focusing on it. Staring into space during a boring flight is to be avoided because it can trigger space myopia.

Hearing 7

Three hours cruising along at 4,500 feet in my homebuilt was exhilarating. This is real flying, I thought. I even opened up the window to smell the fresh air rushing by my face. Because I was flying VFR over the plains, I didn't need to talk to anyone. Then I landed, feeling great. My son came over to me from the hangar. I could see his lips moving as he got closer, but I couldn't hear anything. I also became aware that the ringing in my ears was worse than usual. In the car on the way home, I had to turn up the volume on the radio. My son commented that I used to yell at him to turn the volume down on his stereo, but here I was doing the same in the car. Then it dawned on me. I really couldn't hear well. My doctor confirmed this using an audiometer—it was the first hearing test I'd had for years. I not only had a permanent hearing loss but also it was significantly worse than before. Now I was wondering if I could pass my FAA medical.

HEARING IS SECOND only to vision as an important physiological sense in flight. What and how well you hear dictates your ability to communicate. It allows you to detect audible changes in engine sounds, the flow of air over the airframe, and subtle changes in the sounds of gyros. Unexpected sounds can alert you to possible problems. The source of sounds assists in maintaining situation awareness. The absence of expected sounds during flight operations can tip you off to potential failure.

Loss of hearing can be disabling, depending on the severity of the loss. The sad irony is that virtually all high-frequency loss of hearing is due to noise exposure. Because you can easily protect yourself from noise, there is no reason to suffer the most common cause of hearing loss in aviation.

Anatomy and Physiology of the Ear

Anatomically your ear is divided into outer, middle, and inner parts. These parts take sound waves (an energy source) from outside your body, concentrate them, and finally send them for your brain to interpret. Hearing is your perception of sound energy as well as the ability to discriminate the origin of the sound (Fig. 7-1).

Outer Ear

The outer ear includes the auricle, the external canal and the eardrum. Sound waves are picked up, directed, and focused down the canal to the eardrum by the auricle. The eardrum is set into motion by the force of the sound waves, moving back and forth with each wave.

Anything that obstructs this transmission of wave energy through the air diminishes or distorts the energy necessary to move your eardrum. Ear wax, which everyone makes in varying amounts, is the most common obstruction. By the way, don't try to remove ear wax plugs with a Q-tip—it will only push the plug farther into the ear.

Fig. 7-1 The ear is divided into the inner, middle, and outer parts.

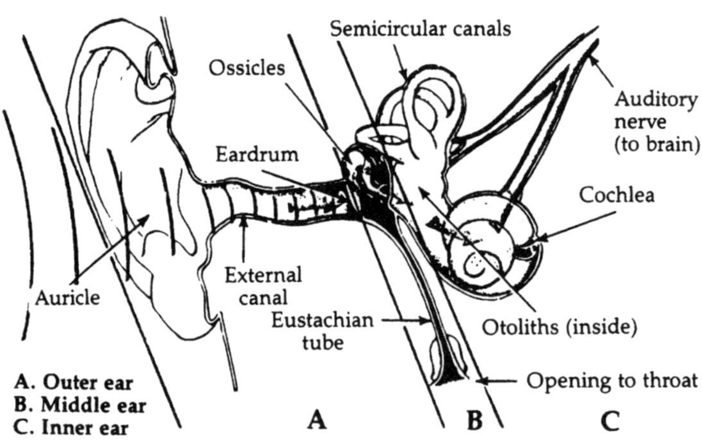

The eardrum also is affected by infection, swelling from an ear block, scarring from an old infection, or even perforation, each impairing the transfer of sound energy into mechanical energy.

Middle Ear

Your middle ear is an air-filled cavity, with pressure equal to the air around you on both sides of the eardrum. Within this cavity is a chain of three tiny bones called ossicles that are set into motion by the vibration of the eardrum. This process transforms airwave energy into mechanical energy. This mechanical energy then proceeds to the cochlea of the inner ear as the signal continues its journey toward your brain.

Interference in the motion of the ossicles, especially at their joints, is very common. This interference causes a diminished or distorted signal transmission. Some sources of interference are fluid within the middle ear, inflammation or stiffening of the joints between the bones, calcification of the joints, and physical dislocation. The most common problems occur with a middle-ear infection (often with fluid), and an ear block from trapped gas.

Inner Ear

Your inner ear contains the cochlea, the otolith organ, and semicircular canals. The cochlea, which resembles a seashell, converts the mechanical energy of ossicle movements into nerve impulses. These nerve impulses are then transmitted to your brain for interpretation.

The ossicles are attached to a flexible window in the cochlea that moves the fluid behind the window.

The cochlea is filled with fluid and the inner walls are lined with thousands of hairlike receptors that move as the fluid moves. The movement of the hairs is similar to the movement of tall grass in a field as the wind blows or to the movement of weeds in a lake, bending as waves or currents move over them. Movement of each hair stimulates the nerve ending at its base to produce an electrical impulse. This impulse is then transmitted through the cochlear (also called the acoustic or auditory) nerve to your brain.

This effect can easily be demonstrated by moving your right hand over your left arm close enough to touch the hairs but not touching the skin. Just as the movement of your arm hair causes nerve impulses to be generated, allowing you to feel movement, so does the movement of the hairs within your cochlea allow you to hear.

A Team Effort

The parts of your ear work as a team to let you hear the sounds around you. As the tower controller calls out, "Cessna one three seven foxtrot alpha, clear for takeoff one three right," what actually happened? The controller's voice was broadcast by your outer ear as airwaves were channeled down your ear canal to the eardrum. The airwaves caused the eardrum to move, which in turn caused your ossicles to move. The eardrum translates the airwave energy to mechanical energy wherein the ossicles act as a type of mechanical amplifier to accentuate the energy before it reaches the cochlea. The cochlea transforms the mechanical energy from the ossicles to electrical energy in the form of nerve impulses. These nerve impulses are then transmitted to your brain for final interpretation. Your perception of this sequence of sounds (words) is to taxi onto the runway, advance the throttle, and takeoff. Thus, you heard and understood what was said to you. If any part of your hearing system becomes injured, your perception of this same sequence might require you to say, "Tower, say again for Cessna one three seven foxtrot alpha."

Hearing loss due to nerve damage (e.g., by infection or injury) involves the cochlear nerve. Hearing loss due to noise involves the hairs in the cochlea. It's like walking on wet grass and looking at your footsteps that you left behind. Like the grass, most hair cells will repair themselves given enough time. With repeated abuse, however, both the grass and the hairs will be permanently damaged.

Tinnitus or ringing in the ears is common and is a result of some degree of insult or damage to the cochlear nerve. Tinnitus also is often associated with noise exposure. In most cases, common tinnitus is normal and nothing needs to be done about it.

Surrounded by Sound

Sound is defined in the dictionary as that energy which is heard, resulting from stimulation of auditory nerves by vibrations of the ear parts described previously. Sound is a form of wave energy, like electricity, light, and microwaves. They follow the same physical laws as any other energy wave.

Physical Properties of Sound

There are three measurable, objective properties with all sound, whether characterized as useful sound or as noise. How you perceive and interpret the meaning of these physical signals is subjective and ranges from indifference, through your inability to detect sound efficiently, to keen awareness of the cues and their role in flight.

Frequency

Like other wave energy, frequency refers to the number of wave cycles (or oscillations) per second (CPS), also called Hertz or Hz. There is a very large range of frequencies for which mechanical waves can be generated, sound waves being confined to the range that can stimulate your ear and brain to the sensation of hearing. This range is between 20 and 20,000 Hz and is called the *audible range*. Frequencies below and above this range are called *infrasonic* and *ultrasonic* waves, respectively. A pure tone is a single frequency without harmonics or other interference.

Intensity

Intensity describes the loudness of the sound, and intensity can be measured. Because it defines a physical property of energy, this measurement is directly related to how well you hear or interpret a certain frequency or combination of frequencies. It is this intensity at individual frequencies that is being tested by the audiometer. The unit of measure for intensity is the decibel (dB) (Fig. 7-2), which is 10 times the loudness of a base sound. Because the ability of your ear to distinguish differences in loudness decreases as intensity increases, the bel scale is logarithmic; each unit is 10 times as great as the preceding one. By definition, the decibel is the relative difference in power between signals, equal to 10 times the common logarithm of the ratio of the two levels. Thus, sound levels are measured against one defined level, which is 1 bel or 10 dB.

For example, a whisper generates an energy that corresponds to the reference 10-dB level. A departing jet generates 10 billion times the amount of energy as the whisper. Therefore, to find the decibel level you would first take the common logarithm of 10 billion, which is 10 or 10 zeroes, then multiply by 10, which yields 100. The departing jet therefore generates a 100-dB sound level. You don't have to understand the math but at least the example demonstrates the origin of the numbers and the relative intensity. A general rule of thumb that I once learned was that for your ear to be able to detect any increase in intensity, the sound level has to increase by 2 dB. Intensities greater than 130 dB are physically painful.

Fig. 7-2 The decibel scale versus sound intensity.

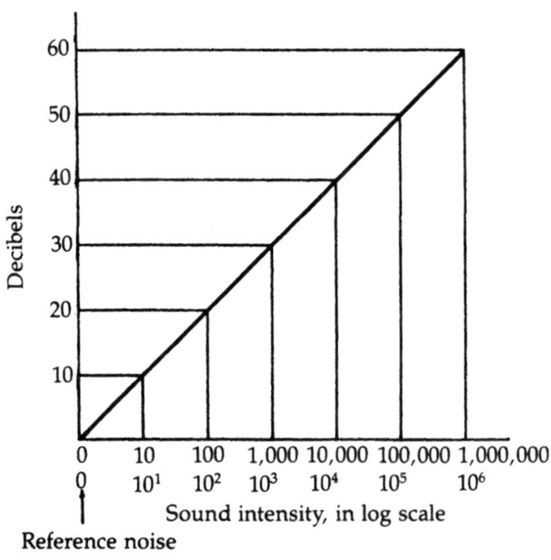

Duration

How long your ear is exposed to a sound determines how well you hear that sound and contributes to your interpretation of its importance (Fig. 7-3). Duration also determines the level of potential risk of injury to your ears. Because sound is energy, it follows that short periods of intense sound are potentially physically detrimental to your hearing. Likewise, the same degree of damage can occur with less intense sounds but for longer periods of time. Therefore, the risk of potential damage to your hearing is not only related to how intense the sound is but also to its duration. It is time related.

Conversational Range

There are three major reasons for your wanting to be able to interpret sounds as they reach your ear. The first is to interpret the sounds of flight: the sound of the engine, the wind over the airframe, and any changes to these sounds that could tip you off as to potential problems. The second is to orient yourself relative to the source of sounds. The third, of course, is to communicate. Although your ear can detect a wide range of frequencies, which enhances the first need, the only frequencies necessary for you to hear to participate in normal conversation are in the conversational range, or 500 to 3,000 Hz. Above and below this range, the sensitivity of your ear decreases rapidly.

Most communication systems in aircraft are not high fidelity because they only operate in the conversational range

Fig. 7-3 Allowable noise exposure.

Exposure duration per day (hours)	Maximum exposure level (dBA)
8	85
6	87
4	90
3	92
2	95
1 1/2	97
1	100
1/2	105
1/4 (ceiling)	110 or less

(500 to 3,000 Hz). Consequently, this is the range most carefully monitored by the FAA in its medical evaluations. Specific intensity (dB) levels at 500, 1,000, 2,000, and 3,000 Hz are one of the few-stated, specific FAA standards.

Definition of Noise

Any sound that you perceive as being too loud, disagreeable, or distracting is considered noise. This interpretation is rather subjective because what you hear as noise may be an important cue to someone else. Regardless, noise still implies sounds that need to be filtered out.

There are two types of noise: steady state and impulse. Steady state noise is what you encounter when you are in or around an operating aircraft, most often during flight. Duration of exposure becomes important in steady state noise because there is a direct correlation to intensity, duration, and amount of damage.

Impulse noise is noise that could be produced by a backfiring engine, switching to a radio that is already turned up to full volume, or other short-term (often lasting only a few milliseconds) but loud (high dB level) sounds, such as gunshots. Often these sounds come as a surprise and there is no way to anticipate the need for added protection.

At the very least, noise is annoying and distracting to you in flight and can cause serious interference with your concentration, communication, and overall performance.

A physiological effect of noise on your entire body, that is often overlooked, is fatigue. Noise, as a form of energy, acts directly on your body as well as on your hearing; therefore, it is more than just an annoyance. Other nonauditory effects of noise include interference with sleep and rest and the proprioceptive system, and other subjective symptoms such as nausea, disorientation, headaches, and general irritability.

Another result of noise exposure is tinnitus. Each of us has some degree of ringing and it would be very noticeable in a quiet room with no background noise. There are very few places without at least some noise (e.g., from circulating air, outside noise of traffic, wind, clocks, etc). Even the drone of the cooling fan in computers and radios is a constant source of noise. Background noise is something that we all learn to tune out. You normally don't notice how much noise you are exposed to until it stops. Tinnitus is more noticeable after exposure to noise, but tends to diminish over time. With significant noise-induced hearing loss, however, increased tinnitus is common. There is no cure for tinnitus. Trying to ignore the ringing is the best solution.

The only accurate way of monitoring the effect noise is having on your hearing is through audiometric testing. Only in this way can you be sure of a lack of damage or impairment.

Perception of Sound

The hearing apparatus within your body provides you with a multitude of valuable signals and cues. The properly functioning ear can determine the origin of a sound, whether above or below, in front, back or to the side of your body.

Your ear is always on. You know this because, for example, loud or abnormal sounds wake you if you are asleep. And most individuals have the ability to filter out the unimportant and tune in the important sounds. You can pick out your call sign among all the other conversations on a busy radio frequency, even if you are concentrating on some other activity. This may not come automatically but with training and most of all, experience, you learn.

If your ear can detect its full frequency range of sounds at low levels of intensity, a vast amount of cues opens up to you for use in situation awareness, often unconsciously. You could, for example, detect a change in airspeed without looking at the gauges. This type of perception comes only from training, experience, familiarity with the aircraft, and a well-functioning pair of ears.

Even when surrounded by noise, your ears and brain can discriminate important sounds from unimportant noise, providing the noise isn't overpowering. The healthy ear can detect faint sounds, especially spoken communications, under a variety of interfering conditions (e.g., noise, thermal extremes, distractions, and multiple activities occurring at the same time). Similarly, many situations interfere with your ability to interpret the sounds around you, including fatigue, hypoxia, stress, and motivational factors, to name a few.

Measurements of Hearing

Because sound is a form of energy, it can be quantified. By sending a pure tone on a specific frequency and at a specific intensity to your ear, the perception of that sound can be identified for all frequencies. This testing is done using an audiometer. The ideal setting is for you to be in a soundproof booth wearing a headset to listen to each tone. For screening purposes, a good headset in a quiet room will do the job.

All FAA exams require testing to be done on your hearing. A common method is the whispered voice test, now called a voice test or conversation test. This is a poor substitute for the audiometer because a voice test cannot quantify nor identify the frequency at which a hearing loss may be present. Only with an audiometer can a reliable result be achieved.

The test results from an audiometer are the audiograms that describe a curve for each ear (Fig. 7-4). Normal hearing should be a straight line in the 5 to 10 dB range. Some variations from normal are acceptable, but any frequency with a loss of greater than 20 dB is considered significant and needs to be further evaluated, especially if it's a change within the last year.

Over time, by comparing audiograms, you and your FAA examiner can see shifts that may be occurring. If high frequencies are being affected, then you need to look at getting better hearing protection. A baseline audiogram is very important. Without this audiogram, you have no way of gauging future test results to see if there are any changes.

Noise and Hearing Loss

There are several issues involved with noise causing hearing loss. The first is for you to recognize that noise is present everywhere and is potentially detrimental, both in performance and in the health of your ear and hearing system. The next is to protect your ears from noise by wearing appropriate hearing protection. The third is to be part of an ongoing hearing conservation program with annual monitoring of hearing abilities and retraining in noise avoidance.

Fig. 7-4 Pilots should get regular audiograms.

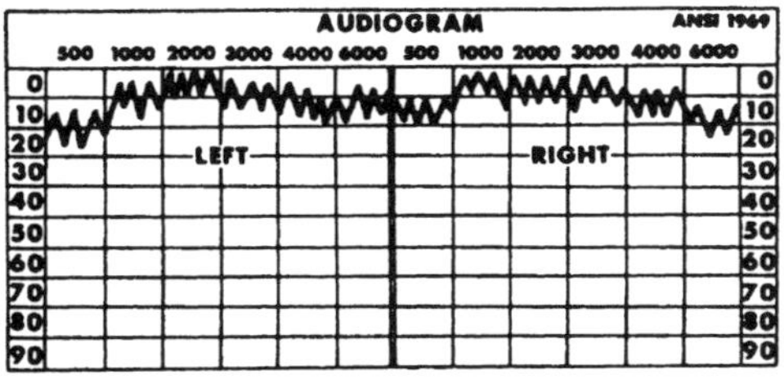

Normal hearing: Has no difficulty with faint speech and little difficulty with speech in a noisy background.

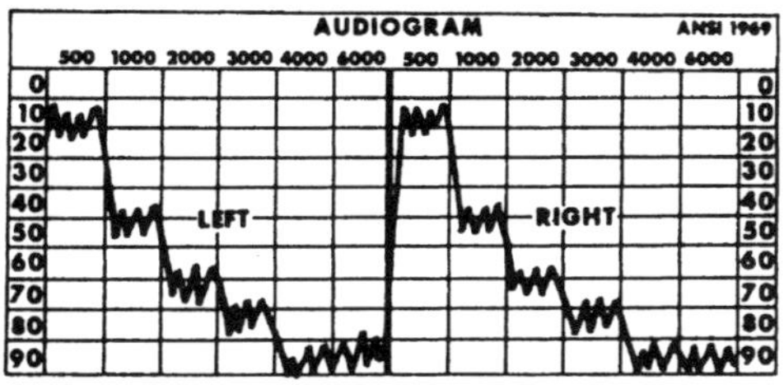

Mild hearing loss: Has some difficulty with speech in a noisy background, ringing sensation (tinnitus) might be present, some combat sounds might not be detected, e.g., clipping barbed wire, dog tags rattling, loose cartriges in pocket, man walking through grass.

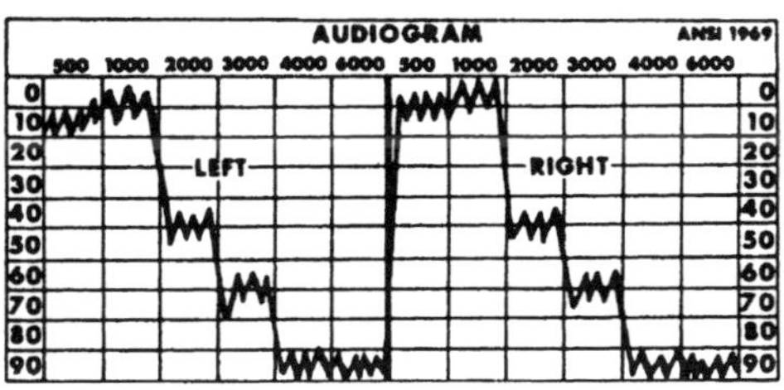

Moderate hearing loss: Has difficulty with normal speech, ringing sensation (tinnitus), may combat sounds not detected, possible hearing aid candidate.

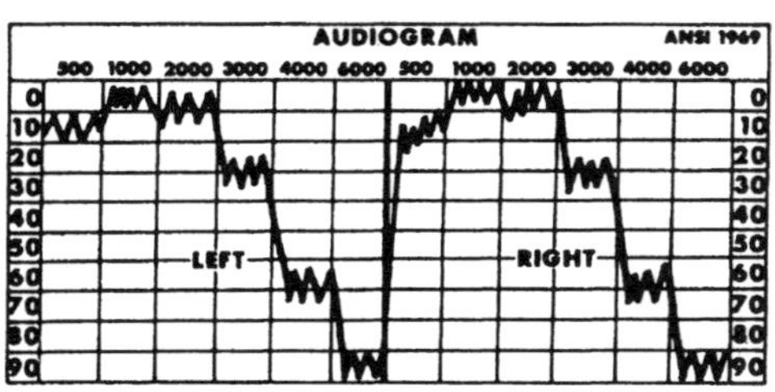

Severe hearing loss: Has difficulty even with loud speech, ringing sensation (tinnitus), needs hearing aid, auditory training, lip reading, speech conservation and speech correction.

Hearing Loss

Noise is recognized as the most common cause of high-frequency hearing loss. There are other causes of general hearing loss, however, some of which are uncontrollable.

Alcohol	Allergy
Arthritis	Aspirin
Burns	Cancer
Chicken pox	Cholesteatoma
Colds	Diabetes
Ear infection	Head injury
Heredity	Hypertension
Hypothyroidism	Influenza
Measles	Meniere's disease
Meningitis	Mononucleosis
Mumps	Otosclerosis
Pneumonia	Polyps
Quinine	Thrombosis
Toxins	Tumors

Sources of Noise

Airplanes and airport ramps are some of the noisiest environments in which you could work. You also are exposed to sounds varying from the continuous low-level noise of a cross-country flight to short periods of engine runups on the ramp. In addition, there is noise associated with many activities not related to aviation in each of our lives such as hobbies, mowing the lawn, downtown traffic, etc.

Occupational Safety and Health Administration (OSHA) has determined certain levels of noise for many different events and activities (Fig. 7-5). Each is time weighted, which means that damage is done with lower levels for longer periods of time. For example, 8 hours of exposure to noise levels of 90 dB is as harmful as 2 hours at 100 dB. It is surprising how much energy there is in some sources. Rock concert's sound reaches 120-dB levels and walking around with headsets at full volume

Fig. 7-5 OSHA standards for noise exposure.

Decibels (In dB/A)	Sounds
0	Threshold of hearing for young ears at 1,000 Hz
20	Whisper at 5 feet
30	Broadcasting studio speech
30–40	Country residence
40–60	Noisy home or typical office
50–70	Normal conversation
60–80	Noisy office, average street noise, average radio
70–80	Automobiles at 20 feet
90	OSHA standard for 8 hours work
80–100	Loud street noise
90–100	Public address system
100	OSHA standard for 2 hours work
100–110	Power lawn mower
105	OSHA standard for 1 hour work
100–120	Thunder, snowmobile
110	OSHA standard for ½ hour work
115	Rock concert
130	Pain threshold for humans
140–160	Jet engine
167	Saturn V rocket

focuses virtually all that energy right into the ear, much like a megaphone.

Airplanes are not quiet to say the least. Many small airplanes with reciprocating engines are very noisy. Prop noise ranges from 90 to 115 dB. Even in the passenger cabin of airliners, there are noise levels that are harmful if you are exposed to them over extended periods of time. As a general rule, anytime you must raise your voice to be heard by someone next to you, you are in a noisy environment. Furthermore, for every 4- or 5-dB increase in sound above 85 dB, the safe time limit for exposure is cut in half.

Noise-Induced Hearing Loss

Noise not only causes interference of communication but also causes permanent high-frequency hearing loss. It is an insidious change, taking years to develop significant loss. Hearing aids do not help noise-induced hearing loss. Thus, noise alone can reduce hearing over the years and there is nothing you can do to reverse the process—it's permanent! You won't know there is a change occurring over time unless you check for it. Like so many other issues in medicine, the best and only treatment is recognition and prevention.

Many pilots have experienced the temporary loss of hearing after a long trip in a noisy airplane. There are stories about people who start their cars for the ride home and then restart the engine because they cannot hear the engine running. This sort of hearing loss reverses in a few days but is also an indication that there was a significant noise exposure that eventually could lead to a permanent loss.

Threshold Shift

As exposure to noise persists, without protection, there is an increasing risk of hearing being impaired, especially in the higher frequencies. You may not even notice this threshold shift as there is no change in your perception of sound. And there is no pain to warn you. There is no way for you to compare your hearing to normal or what is expected from previous perceptions of sounds without testing.

Because this change occurs over several years, it occurs without you noticing until there is extensive hearing loss. As the loss becomes even more severe, speech recognition becomes difficult if not impossible, especially when background noise is present that is at a dB level equal to the hearing loss.

Threshold shifts can be temporary as when you are subjected to short periods of sound infrequently. With continuous exposure (e.g., months) to even moderate noise, this threshold shift becomes more and more permanent. Only monitoring and comparing results of audiograms alerts you to any shifts.

Common Misconceptions about Noise

1. Noise-induced hearing loss can be cured.
Once a hearing loss due to noise becomes permanent, there is very little the doctors can do for you.

2. I can tell when my hearing is getting bad.
Not necessarily. Although some hearing losses occur from a single high-noise exposure, most occur so gradually that you can't tell until it's too late.

3. Ear defenders (earplugs, headsets) are a safety hazard.
In a hazardous noise field, you can distinguish a warning shout or other sound ***better*** *with ear defenders on.*

4. Headsets provide much better ear protection than earplugs.
Each provides approximately the same noise attenuation. Wearing both in very noisy conditions is the best combination.

5. Molded ear pieces offer the best protection, and I can hear the radio better.
You may hear the radio better, but in a noisy cockpit there is very little noise attenuation. Turning the volume up to overcome the background noise could put too much energy against the eardrum.

Other Types of Hearing Loss

Although noise is the greatest and most common cause of hearing loss, especially among pilots and other aircrew, there are other causes. Age, health, and individual sensitivity increase loss. In addition, the following also are found when tested with proper equipment and techniques.

Conductive

When there is some defect or impediment of sound transmission from the external ear to the inner ear, conductive loss is identified. Such a loss involves all frequencies, not just high frequencies. Such situations develop from wax buildup, fluid in the middle ear from infections, ear block, or allergies and colds. Also, the ossicles can become calcified around their joints similar to what can happen to any joint in the body. Most of these situations are treatable and hearing can be restored.

Sensorineural

Sensorineural hearing loss occurs when the hair cells of the cochlea are damaged or inflamed. This can occur from noise exposure as well as from age or infection. Tumors have been known to cause sensineural hearing loss. Because the lower frequencies also are affected, this is a clue that hearing loss is more than just noise related. This type of hearing loss often is not curable.

Conservation of Hearing

It bears repeating. The only way to cope with noise and hearing loss is through identification, prevention, and conservation of the hearing you already have (or have left after suffering a loss). This program—required in the military of everyone on flying status—should be adopted by you, the individual pilot. Only you can be responsible for the protection of your hearing and you are the only one to blame if preventable hearing loss develops.

A successful program consists of three phases. The first is to define a baseline audiogram. If you have never had an audiogram, then get one as soon as possible. If your AME doesn't do audiograms, seek out one who does or see an audiologist (usually listed in the local Yellow Pages of the phone book).

The next phase is to structure a monitoring program. The ideal is to have your FAA exams done by an AME who already does audiograms as part of his or her FAA medical exam. Otherwise, an annual audiogram from the audiologist is important. Keep a copy of the audiogram in your personal files to track any shifts.

The final phase is to wear hearing protection in all noisy areas, especially at work. Noise-induced hearing loss is easy to prevent, if you wear protection. Many of the newer headsets have adequate noise attenuation. Of utmost importance with any headset is the seal between the ear cups and your ears. If that seal is broken or interrupted, noise can enter your ears.

The simplest and least expensive type of protection is the common moldable foam type of earplug. You use this type by rolling it into a tube, inserting it into the ear canal and holding it there until it expands and stays in place. These plugs are very effective. The more expensive earplugs offer little or no better protection. The inexpensive plugs can be purchased by the dozen, so you can always have them available. Keep them in your aircraft, your flight bag, at home, or in the passenger section, and keep extras in your flight suit or map case. Plain cotton or tissue is useless because it does not block the damaging frequencies.

Custom-molded ear pieces, which also are used for communication, are controversial. Many pilots swear by them, others find them uncomfortable and ineffective. Be sure to have the manufacturer quantify the amount of attenuation before purchasing the ear pieces and compare their performance and attenuation standards to a traditional headset.

A common question on the use of earplugs is, What is their effect on hearing what you want to hear—is there a reduction in communication? Ear defenders and other hearing protection all do the same thing. If the ambient noise level is such that you can't hear or communicate without shouting, then protection is necessary to block out the ambient noise. The intent is to be able to maintain clarity of speech and to detect changes in the sounds of flight. Noise is an interference and can be blocked out with earplugs without sacrificing the needed sounds.

The other equally important reason to wear hearing protection is to prevent permanent hearing loss and other associated symptoms, such as fatigue. Once you are in the habit of wearing earplugs or attenuating headsets, there is no compromise to communication.

Sleep, Jet Lag, and Fatigue 8

It was one of those days where nothing went as planned. There was a 2-hour delay in clearance for departure. All we could do was sit it out. The poor night's sleep in the noisy motel was catching up with me. The three cups of coffee I drank helped but I still wasn't very alert by the time we took off. At cruise, which was boringly uneventful, I found myself missing ATC calls. Maybe it was because of the noise in the cockpit, which seemed to be especially noticeable on this trip. And to add to the misery, I knew I was coming down with the flu—the rest of my family was just getting over it. We were only a couple of hours into the flight and I was beat, already really fatigued, but I couldn't understand why when all I was doing was sitting in the cockpit.

PROBABLY THE MOST frequently experienced human factor and physiological situation is fatigue. Most physiological events—noise, hypoxia, dehydration, temperature extremes, etc.—include fatigue as a symptom. Lack of sleep (or sleep debt) and jet lag are commonly considered the most frequent causes of fatigue. There are other causes and these will be discussed, but lack of restful sleep is a cornerstone and may create a cumulative problem with these other sources.

Aviation itself is often the source of virtually all causes of fatigue. This mandates that you, the pilot or flight attendant, must be familiar with the various causes of fatigue and their related symptoms. Some causes cannot be controlled (e.g., length of flight, circadian changes, inadequate inflight nutrition, etc.). But if you are knowledgeable you can cope with these situations by being better prepared, avoiding controllable causes of fatigue, and maintaining a high index of suspicion of your own performance and that of your other crewmembers in potentially fatiguing situations.

Sleep

A basic understanding of the sleep process is important, but even more important is how you deal with the variations in your work and rest requirements.

Anatomy of Sleep

Everyone has the same basic stages of sleep. There are individual variations, however, as to the length and depth of each stage, the number of hours of sleep needed in a 24-hour cycle, and how the benefits of sleep are used.

Stages of Sleep

Essentially, there are four stages of sleep that define the depth of consciousness (or sleep) (Fig. 8-1). The deeper you sleep, the more your body and mind are truly at rest. These four stages occur in a series of cycles over the period of sleep, occurring about every 90 to 100 minutes. Associated with these stages is another stage called *rapid eye movement (REM) sleep*. REM sleep often occurs as you return to the first stage of sleep and just before going back into the next cycle. The other four stages of sleep are called *non-REM sleep*.

Stage 1: Stage 1 sleep encompasses the time between your being awake and when you begin to become drowsy. Your brain waves begin to slow down, your body relaxes, body temperature, respiration, and pulse rate decrease. Some people notice (or see in others) a quick jerking movement of muscles that is an indication of a change in the brain activity. When this happens it may wake you, but you quickly return to sleep. This stage lasts only from 1 to 10 minutes, depending on how fast you fall asleep.

Stage 2: During this stage your brain activity increases for a time, with many short bursts of thoughts and memories. Your muscles become more relaxed, body functions slow, and your breathing becomes steady. If you were to be awakened during this stage, you may deny that you were asleep when in fact you were. This stage lasts about 10 minutes before entering into the third stage.

Fig. 8-1 Anatomy of sleep.

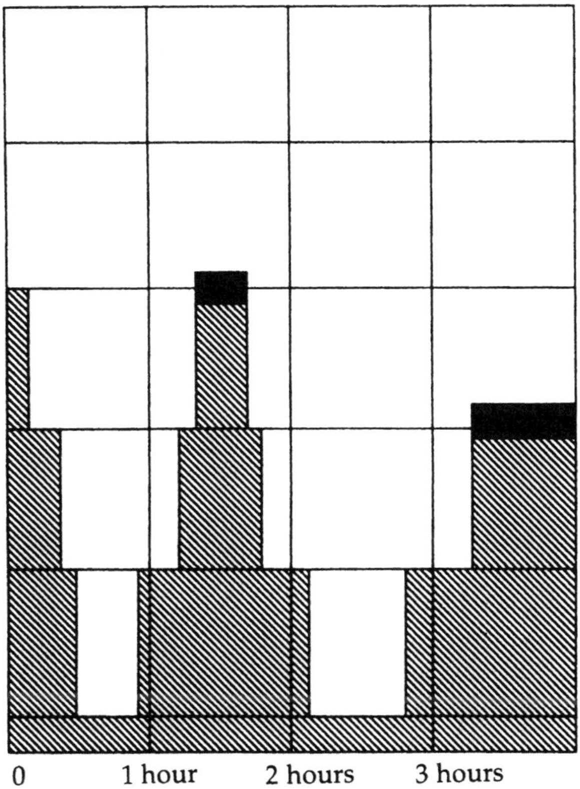

Stage 3: Continued relaxation occurs during stage 3 with your respiration and pulse rate becoming even slower. Your body is almost totally at rest and it would be difficult for someone to wake you during this stage. If awakened, you will not feel rested and may actually feel more tired. It is also sometimes called a transitional stage and lasts for about 5 minutes.

Stage 4: This stage is when the deepest part of sleep occurs. Your body is completely relaxed and your brain activity is slow. You could be considered unconscious and you would be very difficult to arouse. If you did awake, for any reason, you would be very groggy, probably incapacitated for several minutes, and end up with a disturbed sleep cycle or sleep inertia. This stage lasts from about 30 to 45 minutes, the longest period of the cycle. It is during this stage of sleep that, if broken, creates more of a problem to you than if no sleep had occurred. Naps, therefore, must be timed so that you do not reach stage 4 sleep or spend little time there.

REM Sleep: Concurrent with the four stages of sleep, REM occurs about 90 minutes after you fall asleep. In REM sleep, your pulse rate and blood pressure fluctuate, larger muscles remain relaxed but smaller muscles (e.g., in the fingers and toes) may twitch, and, of course, your eyes are moving rapidly even while asleep. This REM stage coincides with the cycle returning to stage 1 and can last for 10 minutes before the cycle moves to stage 2. As each cycle repeats (about every 90 minutes), less time is spent in stages 3 and 4 and more in REM. Therefore, most of your deep sleep occurs early in the total sleep period and REM occupies more of the sleep cycle during the end of the sleep.

Anything that interferes with your REM sleep (e.g., alcohol, drugs, stress, or being wakened during this stage by any strange noise) results in nonproductive sleep and is not restful. A good night's sleep implies an uninterrupted series of non-REM stages and a complete REM stage. Thus, you need to complete at least one full sleep cycle uninterrupted.

As you get older you tend to awaken when you complete the cycle just as you return to stage one and enter REM sleep. For a brief moment you are conscious of being awake, possibly feel that you haven't even been asleep, but then return to the next cycle of sleep. This frequent awakening as you become older is not abnormal and is not an indication of true insomnia.

Variations on Normal Sleep

There are individual changes to a typical sleep cycle. Some people are able to feel rested and function normally with as little as 3 to 5 hours of sleep per day. Others require more than 8 hours. The 8-hour norm of sleep is universal but you must determine your own optimum amount of restful sleep.

Some people can easily fall asleep if just given the opportunity, even in noisy, uncomfortable locations. They are able to take quick "cat naps" and keep ahead of their sleep needs. Others find it very difficult to quickly get to sleep, even under ideal conditions. Again, this can be a normal variation and not something that is easily changed. Nor should it be, unless you have true insomnia, which will be discussed later. You should avoid quick fixes to try to change a sleep habit that is normal for you.

Everyone's sleep cycle is determined by his or her own circadian rhythm. The cycle of sleep is one of the most important rhythms and it can be easily disrupted if your sleep cycle, when it occurs, is changed as in jet lag. Along with this internal clock, there is also a variation from your rhythm compared with someone else's. Some people are larks, or morning people. They awake early, ready to go, and alert to the world around them, but they also tend to begin to lose that energy about mid-afternoon. The owl or night person, in contrast, takes hours to get going after awakening, with their full energy available about mid-afternoon and lasting well into the evening. Larks go to bed much earlier than owls.

Sleep Disorders

When your sleep is disrupted or inadequate (not restful), sleep debt occurs. This is also called *insomnia*. There are three different categories of insomnia. The most common and least important is the transient kind, which lasts for only a few nights. This kind of insomnia is often a result of excitement (e.g., just got a major raise in salary), the jitters (e.g., anticipating an upgrade checkride you don't feel ready for), and other reasons we have all experienced that keep us from getting to sleep. The mind just won't let you relax or tune out your thoughts. Once the situation causing this form of insomnia is resolved, sleep patterns quickly return to normal.

Acute or short-term insomnia results from longer-lasting stress (e.g., your company may be sold) or illness (e.g., a bad case of flu). It's also frequent in extended days and nights on long trips, staying at a variety of less-than-favorable sleeping facilities. These situations usually resolve themselves in a few days and no longer interfere with sleep, and your cycles return to normal. You may actually lose sleep but you can recover after several good nights of restful sleep. Depending on the amount of sleep loss, your health, age, and other factors, however, it may take you longer to recover than you would expect. Unless acute insomnia persists, it's not wise to have unrealistic expectations of a sleep pattern that never changes.

Chronic insomnia is more serious and comes from continuing sources of sleep deprivation. This can last for days, weeks, or even months. The most common cause in the general public is serious, unresolved stress and illness. For you, the aircrew member, it's a combination of several factors, including unresolved stress. Some have observed that it's not so much the lack of sleep as much as *when* the sleep is allowed to occur in a 24-hour period. Long-haul trips, day after day of flight instruction, and frequent night flights are all inherent in aviation. Some people can adapt, others can't. If you can't and you feel you are never fully rested, then changes must be made. Insomnia is a symptom and the cause of your insomnia is the prime concern. Therefore, take care of the cause first without focusing on trying to treat the symptom. Chronic insomnia usually needs the help of your doctor.

Factors Affecting Sleep

Most aircrew are familiar with what interferes with a good sleep. The first factors to be considered are noisy rooms or sleeping quarters, uncomfortable beds, hot or cold temperatures, too much light, and other environmental factors, often beyond your control. Wearing earplugs can keep out noise, putting a blanket over a window can shut out the light, and extra blankets can make the bed more comfortable. There are a variety of other creative ways to isolate yourself from the discomforts of the new sleeping environment.

Other controllable factors are self-imposed stresses such as too much caffeine from any source (e.g., coffee, tea, colas, cocoa, some OTC drugs). Nicotine is another stimulant that can interfere with restful sleep. Alcohol interferes with REM sleep and many believe that if REM sleep is disrupted, then restful sleep is compromised. This effect on sleep can last for several hours after the last drink (and that includes wine and beer if taken in excess). Changes in your circadian rhythms (desynchronosus) also can affect sleep, especially when trying to sleep at times when your body is not ready to sleep. Circadian rythms will be discussed later.

Symptoms of Insomnia

Symptoms of insomnia are similar to those associated with fatigue and will be covered in the section on fatigue. Generally, there is a pronounced decrease in performance, especially in decision-making and fine muscle skills. Motivation to do a good job is diminished, and like with hypoxia, you don't really care. You have lapses in alertness and a tendency to slip into short periods of sleep (micro sleep) and not even be aware that you were asleep. Small errors and mistakes are exaggerated. A major problem is the vicious circle of insomnia—stress from not sleeping well, the fear of being an insomniac—all leading ultimately to poor sleep.

How to Sleep

There are several measures you can take to improve your chances of getting a restful sleep. Try to maintain the same sleep schedule, especially when you are at home. Staying up to watch the late movie and sleeping in late on weekends only confuses your body's rhythms and disrupts sleep. Exercise and keeping in shape is a major factor that allows your body to relax more efficiently and to tolerate factors that could keep you awake. At home, sleep in sound- and light-proof rooms in comfortable conditions.

Stress and thinking about the stress often interfere with your sleep. It's difficult to mentally turn off your concerns and to avoid laying awake considering all the bad things that could happen. At night, alone with your thoughts, these stresses are often out of proportion to reality. Imagination runs rampant. Getting up and writing down your thoughts with some ideas on how to resolve them sometimes helps to break the cycle and allows you to get to sleep. Bear in mind that, as you get older, you tend to enter the wake phase of a sleep cycle during REM. If you begin rehashing and ruminating about these stresses, it will be difficult to slip back into sleep. The counting sheep technique, as well as other similar tips, attempts to break this focus by forcing your mind to think of a mundane event that, in turn, allows the less active mind to return to a sleep stage.

Your diet plays a role in the quality of your sleep. Carbohydrates tend to make you drowsy; therefore foods high in carbohydrates can be eaten before retiring to stimulate sleepiness. Thus, the old-fashioned remedy of warm milk before bedtime has a physiological basis. L-tryptophan, an amino acid found in many carbohydrates, is considered by some to be the sleep inducer. Foods for you to avoid before bedtime (in addition to caffeine and alcohol) are those high in protein and animal fat because they tend to keep you more alert.

OTC sleeping pills are almost always antihistamines. Their side effect of sedation may help you get to sleep but this is not necessarily a restful sleep. Furthermore, the effects can last for hours after you awake because the half-life is so long (see Chapter 5). Antihistamines also have significant side effects in flight, in addition to sedation, which could still be present if you fly shortly after you awake. By reading the label, you will see that the same kinds of chemicals that are used in allergy medications are used in sleeping pills.

Staying Awake

Some of the above-mentioned factors also can be used to keep you from falling asleep. Caffeine is the traditional example, but the timing of intake is important so as not to interfere with sleep when you are ready to sleep. Avoid carbohydrates and sugary foods that are common in the vending machine breakfasts, lunches, and snacks. In addition to the drowsiness common with carbohydrates, hypoglycemia can be a common result if there isn't sufficient fat or protein. Although you may get an energy burst from the sugars, you will ultimately become drowsy. Eat small meals, high in protein; peanuts, for example. Keep active and avoid boring or nonmotivating tasks. Save them for later when you want to sleep. Drink lots of water, and change positions frequently, and even get up and walk around. Anything that keeps you mentally and physically active helps you to stay awake.

Circadian Rhythms

Your body has biological rhythms, at least 300 different kinds, that are periodic relative to the revolution of the earth and to the rising of the sun. Circadian literally means "about a day" and usually represents a 24-hour day. Another term used to describe rhythms is *diurnal*, which means that a cycle occurs within a day.

Human Rhythms

Studies have shown that if you were to be removed completely from any source of time or outside sunlight, your body's rhythms would settle around a cycle of about 25 to 26 hours. You reset your internal clock, which establishes your rhythms, every day by getting up at the same time with the help of an alarm clock, reporting to work at a given time, and more importantly, by exposure to sunlight at these times.

You may have heard the term *biorhythms*. It is an unscientific claim that how you feel and how you act during a day are based on your biorhythm for that day. This is comparable to astrology. There are biological rhythms, which is what I am discussing, but there is no scientific basis for biorhythm predictions.

Circadian rhythms are true rhythms; that is, there are hourly variations for each function that has a rhythm, highs and lows, and steady states. A curve can be plotted for each physiological function that has a rhythm.

Common Human Circadian Rhythms

Probably your most important circadian rhythm is your sleep cycle, which I have just discussed. Many people are able to wake without the help of a clock and others are able to estimate time without a watch. You feel tired and ready for bed at a specific time and you tend to follow that urge. If your cycle is not followed, your body responds with the same symptoms recognized for sleep deprivation and for fatigue in general. In aviation, this is a major problem because you may cross several time zones, which means the sun and the people at the destination are several hours off your own established rhythms for sleep. We are now living in a 24-hour society, with people working every hour of every day. Aircrew are especially affected by this reality.

Weekends at home can result in a miniature change in sleep circadian rhythm. For example, Friday, Saturday, and possibly Sunday night are usually spent staying up until long after your usual bedtime. You add to disrupting your rhythm by sleeping in late on Saturday and possibly Sunday. By Monday morning, the body feels as if it were on the West coast when you really are getting up on the East coast, relatively speaking. The Monday morning blues could be another name for weekend jet lag.

Temperature change is another powerful rhythm that affects performance throughout the day. It reaches its peak about mid-day and then begins to drop off. Night people (owls) peak out toward the end of the day, Larks peak earlier. This variation in circadian temperatures affects and determines your level of activity, feelings, and alertness.

You also have an alertness cycle. That is, there are two periods during a 24-hour period that you are less alert and less in tune with your activities. These lulls in the cycle are when you are most prone to making errors and performing below normal. They occur between 4 and 6 AM and PM. Many major air and road accidents have occurred during these times.

Your appetite is also diurnal. The body expects food at certain times based on how your body is programmed by your own eating habits. If you don't eat at these expected times, your appetite goes away and you may not have the urge to eat for several hours, especially if you are distracted by other activities. Or you may eat a large meal when your body isn't quite ready, subjecting it to additional stress of unexpected energy necessary for metabolism. Your body also expects to have a bowel movement at a certain time. If you don't because you are off schedule, the urge goes away. Over a period of a few days constipation occurs and you may not be aware that you haven't had a bowel movement. Being dehydrated and failing to eat enough fiber on a long trip complicates this problem.

Circadian Rhythms and Jet Lag

When circadian rhythms are disrupted, desynchronosus (jet lag) occurs. When you travel north and south there are no time zone changes. Yet there are fatigue-like symptoms similar to those experienced with traditional jet lag. The reason is that a major source of the symptoms is related to the length of the trip, which is fatiguing in itself. The same added problems of dehydration, hypoxia, sitting for long periods of time, poor nutrition, etc., complicate the symptoms no matter which direction you travel.

There are, obviously, symptoms that are directly related to traveling across several time zones but only because the circadian changes conflict with the destination's sunlight and activities. These symptoms include headache, poor sleep, constipation, disrupted eating habits, vertigo, poor short-term memory, depression, to name a few. There is a general feeling of being out of it. Note that these symptoms are similar to the symptoms associated with fatigue alone. So fatigue and its symptoms are essentially the main symptoms of desynchronosus and obviously they compound your awareness of impairing symptoms.

For most people, traveling west is easier than traveling east. Part of the reason is because when you are headed west you are traveling with the sun. Because the real day for your body is 25 or more hours, there is less of a problem as you gain time moving westward and are exposed to the sun. Unless you are staying for several days or longer, however, you still have to come back east. It's this continuous changing of your physiological rhythms, relative to the sun, that increases the symptoms of fatigue.

Coping with Jet Lag

Studies show that the greatest chance for error occurs between 4 and 6 AM of your current diurnal rhythms (Fig. 8-2). If you now travel to a location where you are expected to perform safely but it is in the middle of the day and 5 AM your body time, then you are at high risk for making errors. This risk decreases as you begin to adapt to the local time.

Pilots and flight attendants, however, rarely stay very long in one place during a trip, no matter how far away from their home station. If you anticipate that you are going to be affected, there are measures that might help you to cope with this change in body rhythms, especially if you are going to be at the same location for several days.

Get into the sun as soon as possible at the final destination.

Jet Lag

Physical Symptoms

- Fatigue
- Digestive difficulty
- Altered kidney and bowel function
- Unusually pronounced reaction to alcohol
- Maladjustment in mood, judgment, and general functional ability

Aviation Factors that Contribute to Physical Symptoms

- Oxygen deficiency
- Warm cabin temperature and low humidity
- Long periods of sitting
- Decreased cabin pressure

Preventive Measures

- Readjust your sleep schedule
- Get a good night's rest the night before departure
- If possible, schedule stopovers instead of straight-through flights when crossing multiple time zones
- Exercise in your seat and move about cabin when possible
- Before departure, adjust your meal schedule gradually to the new time zone
- Try to avoid tension and stress before departure
- Don't overeat and avoid alcohol during the flight

Treatments after Arrival

- Get plenty of sleep
- Drink plenty of fluids
- Eat only food to which you are accustomed at first

Fig. 8-2 Jet lag has an adverse effect on performance.

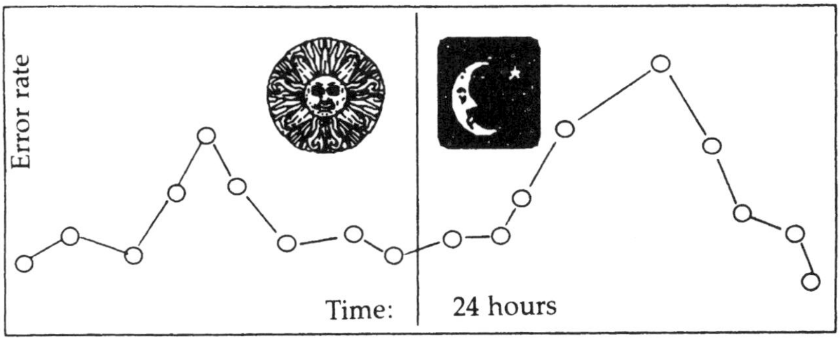

ALL HUMAN FUNCTIONS ebb and flow predictably: the ability to solve math problems, temperature, hormone levels, sensitivity to drugs and pain, oxygen consumption, heart rate and blood pressure and, of course, sleeping and waking. Changing your daily schedule can disrupt this pattern of cycles. Once disrupted, body rhythms readjust at different rates.

AT THE TIME OF THE DAY when your body temperature falls, mental alertness is also depressed. During an all-night trip, your temperature low and mental dip will probably occur between 4 a.m. and 6 a.m.

THIS GRAPH SHOWS how the likelihood of making an error—from simple lapses of attention to falling asleep—varies through the day. At 4 a.m. the chance of error is 60% higher than average. Between 8 and 11 a.m., people are about 25% less likely to err.

The sun is a powerful mental stimulant. Become active and involved with your destination's time zone activities. You need to be familiar with the effects of caffeine and alcohol and to use them in such a way so as not to interfere with alertness and sleep. For example, alcohol or caffeine on arrival interrupts your sleep when you want to sleep. Eat lightly, keeping in mind the sedative effects of carbohydrates. Jet lag diets are of questionable value according to most circadian experts. But there are some basics that are helpful, such as the type of foods to eat and when to eat them plus the other suggestions already mentioned. The timely use of caffeine and alertness enhancers is important.

The better your health and fitness, the better you can tolerate circadian changes and the quicker you can adapt. Increase your fluids, especially water, and minimize the diuretic effects of alcohol and caffeine. Eat plenty of high-fiber foods such as raw vegetables and bran, which also prevent constipation.

Try to rest before a trip, otherwise you are fatigued even before you get there. Wise long-haul pilots watch with knowing glances as their younger crewmates enjoy the nightlife in an exotic new city only to suffer the fatigue of the next day on the leg back. It's tempting to enjoy the layover but the price paid the next day may be too expensive. Save the sightseeing and fancy eating establishments for longer stays.

Fatigue

As I have stated throughout this chapter, fatigue is the common denominator in virtually all symptoms related to deprived sleep and desynchronosus, as well as in many other physiological stresses unique to flying. It is important for you to recognize that many of the causes are occurring at the same time that the symptoms are present. There can be a quick accumulation of causes and effects, often creeping up on you without you being aware. Like hypoxia and alcohol, fatigue is an insidious deterrent to safety, especially because one of its main symptoms is a lack of awareness and a feeling of indifference to its effects.

There are two general kinds of fatigue, acute and chronic. Like sleep, acute fatigue is related to current events and activities and you will recover when the situation resolves itself so you can rest. Chronic fatigue is more serious in that there is a cumulative effect over several months, creating more fatigue without the benefit of adequate recovery. Such fatigue makes your body vulnerable to illness and increased stress, and is a generally unhealthy condition. Treating chronic fatigue often requires the help of a doctor.

Causes of Fatigue

The following are specific causes of fatigue of which you must be aware. You can then self-monitor your performance when these conditions are present and be suspicious of deteriorating performance. Observing your crewmates is also important because they may not know they are impaired.

Lack of Restful Sleep

The key word in sleep is *restful*. It doesn't matter how long or where sleep takes place. If it is not restful, fatigue results. It often becomes a vicious circle. You are so fatigued that you cannot relax because you are still mentally rehashing the day's activities and anticipating the next leg or trip. You are unable to allow sleep to take over and you become more fatigued. Although alcohol may relax you, it disturbs your REM sleep.

Dehydration

Often overlooked as a cause of fatigue, dehydration is a common occurrence in the airplane. Because outside air, which is very dry, is recirculated, the humidity can become less than 10 percent in a matter of minutes. Being dehydrated for hours and periodically for days results in fatigue that may not be noticed. The solution is simply to drink lots of water. By the time you feel thirsty, you are already dehydrated.

Caffeine

Although considered a stimulant and often used to stay awake (an acceptable practice under the right conditions), drinking too much caffeine keeps your body alert, even to the point of being tense. That, coupled with any trip that may require a lot of mental and physical energy (and adrenaline flow), leaves you fatigued when the destination is reached. This is a form of withdrawal and is a significant factor if you are not rested enough for the next flight, whether in a few hours or the next day. The letdown of not having the stimulation of caffeine leads to fatigue.

Noise and Vibration

Most prop-driven aircraft and all helicopters are noisy. Noise is a form of energy that is not well tolerated by your body for long periods of time. This is frequently confirmed when pilots begin to wear earplugs and noise-attenuating headsets and realize that they are not as tired after the trip. Because you can't avoid noise in most aviation situations, fatigue will be a factor unless adequate protection is worn. Vibration is similar to noise except the frequencies are lower in vibration, but it still causes fatigue. Little can be done to prevent vibration but the combination of earplugs or noise-attenuating headsets, along with adequate padding in the aircraft seats, will help prevent fatigue.

Illness

Your body fights illness through its own metabolism. Colds and flu are common and some aircrew tend to go ahead and fly with these illnesses. Flying sick is fatiguing because of the increased energy needed by your body to combat the illness and the effects of the illness itself. Recall how tired and miserable you felt the last time you had the flu or a cold; the symptoms go beyond the cough and sniffles.

Over-the-Counter Medications

Many medications contain antihistamines whose side effect is sedation. The combination with caffeine (often used in these medications to overcome the effects of drowsiness) is fatiguing. Now you are battling not only the illness but also the effects of the treatment used to fight the illness.

Hypoglycemia

Fatigue is the most serious effect of self-imposed stress and often occurs midmorning when the quickie breakfast has been digested. Proper nutrition and prevention is the best way to deal with hypoglycemia. If you are prone to these symptoms, carry some quick energy in the form of snacks, peanuts, or candy. Fatigue from hypoglycemia is slow to develop and you may not relate how you are feeling to being hypoglycemic.

Hypoxia

To many, fatigue is the first sign of being hypoxic. This is a very subjective sign and you may think that fatigue is the result of something else. Working at altitude, whether in the plane or on the ground, causes fatigue but it probably will be more noticeable when you are hypoxic. In any case, everyone feels fatigued when hypoxic.

Impaired Vision

Pilots in general do not like wearing glasses, especially as they get older. Not wearing glasses (and hoping the eyes and brain will sort the out-of-focus images) is fatiguing. Most have heard of eye strain and that is what the eyes are doing, they are being strained by trying to focus. The obvious solution is to wear glasses all the time, even for reading, and to work with adequate lighting.

Thermal Fatigue

Exposure to conditions of excessive heat and cold is a common source of fatigue. Your body is working to maintain its core temperature and this requires calories and other energy sources. The result of exposure to temperature extremes is fatigue, even after temperature control is reached.

Boredom

You have to be physically and mentally active to keep from being bored. Although not directly fatiguing, the feeling of boredom is perceived as fatiguing. Many of the same symptoms are present in fatigue and boredom. Furthermore, if bored and tired, there is no longer the stimulant effect to overcome the resulting fatigue.

Circadian Change

Fatigue is the most common complaint with long-haul trips across time zones. It's the combination of the length of the trip and the desynchronosus.

Skill Fatigue

Skill fatigue is a little-recognized source of fatigue and is the result of demands of persistent concentration with high demands for skill. It does not require high levels of physical activity. With skill fatigue, there is also an operational problem related to your motivation to continue pushing yourself beyond your capabilities. There is a conflict between your ego and your good judgment because of your desire to fly and complete a mission. The result is fatigue, which is not noticed until after the trip and is especially dangerous if there is another trip (or leg) soon after. This is common in emergency medical evacuation where the mission becomes all-important, when flying in minimums for hours with a lot of traffic, or when practicing for a checkride. The flow of adrenaline overcomes, for a time, the impairment of skill fatigue. Remove the stimulus and fatigue takes over.

Unresolved Stress

Unresolved stress is common for everyone. It's been said that nothing is more fatiguing than the eternal hanging on of an uncompleted task. Personal stress that is not resolved drains your body of energy and is often associated with depression, which also is fatiguing or gives the perception of fatigue. Many visits to a doctor for fatigue are secondary to depression or anxiety.

Symptoms of Fatigue

There are a variety of symptoms directly related to fatigue. Hypoxia, for example, has several symptoms similar to those of fatigue. Therefore, there is a cumulative effect of various causes resulting in more pronounced and significant symptoms.

Probably the most important symptom of fatigue, as with hypoxia and lack of sleep, is the feeling of indifference, of settling for less in performance. You are unaware that you are fatigued and allow your personal acceptable tolerances and limits for performance to expand, which allows for mistakes or substandard skills. You simply take more risks.

Other specific fatigue symptoms unique to flightcrew in flight include the following:

Increased Reaction Time

You take longer to react to a change or emergency. Automatic response to any abnormal flight is slowed such as recovery from a tight turn that is losing altitude or recovery from a

Symptoms of Acute Fatigue

- Need for larger stimulus
- Errors in timing
- Loss of accuracy and control smoothness
- Unaware of error accumulation
- Ease of distraction
- Neglect of secondary tasks
- Inattention

stall. More common is your delayed response to ATC's change in a clearance or the recognition of a warning light. The reduced response time has the potential to turn minor problems into major accidents, both in the air and on the ground.

Channelized Thought Processes

As a fatigued crewmember, you tend to concentrate on one thought or activity at a time, rather than several, which is essential in flying. Concentration is also narrowed, and you focus, for example, only on what the weather is ahead and do not plan your approach. You may be focused on issues outside the cockpit, such as an argument at home or the unknown results of your medical evaluation. Flying demands a multitude of thoughts, all processed by the brain in sequence or sometimes instinctively, not requiring active thinking. The mind can only process pieces of information one at a time. Automatic actions are essential in normal flight. The number of separate thoughts that can and should be processed decreases as fatigue gets worse.

Fixation

When you are fixated, you might focus on a single instrument, stare at a blinking warning light on the panel, or listen intently to a strange sound that is not important to the flight. Your instrument scan becomes less efficient and traffic is missed because you are concentrating on some other object. You may stare at something for several minutes and not be aware that you are doing so.

Short-Term Memory Loss

With short-term memory loss, you may quickly forget what ATC's last clearance was and you didn't think to write it down. Or you forgot to change the radio and are calling departure on tower's frequency. You hear a crewmate call for flaps during other activities but being fatigued, you forget, especially if you are distracted. Small talk while fatigued can cause you to forget what you were about to do, even if it was an important task.

Impaired Judgment and Decision Making

If your judgment is impaired, you make dumb mistakes that, although insignificant, can become another link in a growing chain of events leading to an incident or accident. You take chances and shortcuts rather than follow acceptable procedures. You really know better but just don't realize you're messing up.

Easily Distracted

When fatigued, you are easily distracted. For example, you may notice a falling map from the panel and quickly reach for it rather than holding back. A sound or other visual cue away from a scan and for a brief moment becomes more important than the scan itself. You miss an item on the checklist because you are distracted by conversation that is irrelevant to the flight (the sterile cockpit policy helps prevent this but automation has become another distraction).

Sloppy Flying

Your fine motor skills are compromised in sloppy flying and you find yourself holding onto the yoke with your hands rather than your fingers. You lose the fine tuning of your turns and climbs and change of power settings. More importantly, you have to think about what to do rather than flying by using well-learned and instinctual skills. You have to think too long about which direction to turn to change heading, or in what order controls are changed to begin a descent. Much of flying is automatic and habit. Anything that interferes with the smooth performance of these skills impairs you, and you may not notice the problem. Your instrument flying is not precise and there are errors in timing.

Decreased Visual Perception

In decreased visual perception, it takes longer to focus (accommodate) from a distant object to a near object. This becomes especially critical while flying an instrument approach to landing. The scan takes longer because you can't focus well or you may just skip a part of the scan.

Loss of Initiative

You don't really care anymore when you are fatigued and you are unwilling to maintain your expected high level of skill or accuracy. You become passive about your own high standards of flying. You let someone else make an error and won't say anything. You don't speak up when something doesn't look right.

Personality Change
You become more irritable and are easily depressed with minor problems. There is a decreased tolerance to nagging and irritating habits of a crewmate. You are quick to react negatively.

Attitude
You are willing to settle for less and you are not even aware of your change in attitude and performance. And if you are aware, you don't care.

Depression
Even though you may normally have a positive outlook on life, fatigue can cause you to imagine all kinds of scenarios of how things could go wrong. Depression, although short term, can result in a gloomy perception of life. Being fatigued and depressed is a poor combination in flight.

The following is a possible scenario of what could happen to you on a typical flight if you are fatigued. The obvious continuous thread of concern is your fatigue. I wrote this for *Business & Commercial Aviation* magazine in 1991, and suggest that it will help you relate real-world situations to fatigue.

Let's begin the scenario. It's been a long day with several stops. At two of these stopovers, you waited for several hours. Now your ready to start the last leg and you're flying the plane.

You are cleared to taxi and, enroute to the active, you go through the rest of your "before takeoff" checklist. You are transfixed by an emergency vehicle heading across the tarmac to the terminal and as a result of this minor distraction, you miss the command to set flaps. Your copilot has to remind you later on into the list.

At the last minute, tower tells you to "hold your position for landing traffic," which seems a long way off on final. You let tower know about your dissatisfaction of having to wait for traffic that, in your opinion, is a safe distance. You are usually patient in these conditions, but right now you are more irritable and easily annoyed.

You are finally cleared for takeoff on 23 Right and to fly a heading of 210. You forget the clearance and maintain runway heading until ATC reminds you of the 210 heading. Then you call departure on the tower frequency, another lapse in short-term memory.

As you climb out into the clouds you fixate on a flashing yellow light on the annunciator panel, nothing significant, but you also are sliding into a turn as you stare at the light. Your copilot gets you back on your scan after tactfully saying "heading 210."

You finally reach cruising altitude when ATC requests you to turn 30 degrees to the right for traffic, your copilot is asking where the approach plates are, you are trying to trim the altitude hold, and the waypoint light is flashing. Your mental focus is really on the radar, which is showing thunderstorms on the flight path. Only after ATC has to remind you of your heading change do you realize your thoughts were channelized on only one situation—the radar—when you should have been alert to everything.

The rest of the cruise was uneventful, even boring. Your mind is wandering as you go through your scan. You begin to think about the unopened letter from the IRS sitting on your desk, your FAA medical is due next week and your blood pressure is borderline. Your teenage son got his first speeding ticket yesterday. You imagine many undesirable scenarios for each of these situations and you are beginning to scare yourself—you fear you are becoming depressed even though nothing serious has actually happened.

Finally, you're "cleared to descend to 4,000 at pilot's discretion" while still 75 miles out. You begin an immediate descent. Your copilot questions your judgment and wonders that your decision to go down so soon is premature, knowing it's bumpy lower and your passengers are trying to relax. "What difference does it make? Besides, who is in charge anyway!" you snap back.

ATIS reports 1,000 and 1. You chose to fly the ILS by hand. You find yourself chasing the needle, driving with a firm grip on the yoke instead of flying the airplane with a gentle touch. Then your first bounce is hard and your second floats to a mushy touchdown. You think to yourself that you haven't performed such sloppy flying since your were a student. Your final act of frustration is to yell at your copilot for not alerting you to your altitude.

Most of us have been in one or more of these situations. Fatigue is insidious and there is no way to prevent its symptoms.

The degree of impairment, however, is going to be a result of your awareness of and insight into the whole subject of fatigue and avoiding or controlling the myriad of causes that are occurring simultaneously.

Coping with Fatigue

Unfortunately there is often a fine line between acceptable fatigue and fatigue that could seriously impair your abilities. The challenge is that most significant fatigue often occurs well into the flight. How well you recognize your level of fatigue and can overcome the symptoms of fatigue determines how safe you are to fly.

It is ultimately up to you to make the final decision to fly, based on your perception of your tolerance to fatigue. Being healthy, physically fit, and avoiding the causes of fatigue that were mentioned previously are the only practical means of assisting you in determining if you are safe to fly. The next time that you are seriously fatigued and not flying, make a mental note of your level of impairment.

Common Misconceptions about Sleep and Jet Lag

- I know how tired I am.
- I've lost sleep before and I did just fine.
- I'm motivated enough to just push through it.
- Scheduled rest periods allow for required sleep.

Stress Management, Crew Resource Management, and the Safe Crewmember

9

I was preflighting the aircraft for the third and final leg of the trip. I had brought some personal problems onboard the aircraft at the start of the day and it seemed like the stress had been piling up all day long. Bad weather, diversions, sick passengers ... you name it, I had experienced it on this trip. The stress was manifesting itself in the form of headaches, irritability, and worst of all, poor judgment and being distraction. I hated to give up control of the aircraft, but it was obvious to me and I'm sure to my crewmates that we would all be better off if I let the copilot fly the last leg.

Stress

IF YOU HAVE BEEN piloting aircraft for any length of time, whether for pleasure or career interests, chances are you have experienced some stress as an occupational hazard. Time is often the culprit. In an aviation environment, time is a driving force. Multiple tasks must be performed simultaneously to get them all completed. Fuel management is directly related to time. Demands often exceed the time available. This is of major concern in single-pilot operations and in general aviation where one pilot must often make all of the decisions and perform all of the tasks.

Everyone experiences stress to varying degrees, some more than others. In fact, stress is essential in keeping us from becoming complacent. Someone once said that stress is the price paid to be a race horse instead of a plow horse.

Stress, by itself, is not the problem. How you cope with stress, especially unresolved stress, is what can create a problem.

As mentioned, flying airplanes can be stressful. There is much to learn and much to remember. You learn something new every time you fly. You are being continually monitored and checked. You may have high expectations of yourself, often leading to becoming a perfectionist and thus subjecting yourself to unrealistic goals. These unrealistic expectations increase the amount of stress with which you must deal. Stress can be defined as any activity—either self-imposed or by situations beyond your control—to which you are subjected to and to which you have to cope. How you cope determines how you are affected and what degree of impairment is noticed. If stress becomes unmanageable, then a variety of symptoms develop, such as anxiety, unhappiness, and sometimes panic. No one can be free of stress. If you can cope with stress effectively, you actually become a better pilot.

Stress that is not dealt with effectively leads to distress. When you are able to cope, the stress becomes eustress. If you are unable to cope, you become distressed. You respond with a variety of symptoms such as upset stomach, headaches, muscle cramps, and diarrhea, to name a few. The most common symptom is a feeling of fatigue.

Some situations that are commonly seen in pilots and flight attendants under stress are distraction from tasks, inattention to flight activities, preoccupation with insignificant problems, judgment errors, a mind set on only one way to do something, and technical errors. The responsible crewmember who begins to notice these changes in himself or herself now adds these deficiencies to the underlying stress causing the changes. Your high expectations become eroded, which is stressful in itself. Thus, there develops a circle of stressful and often unrealistic perceptions that leads you to be an impaired pilot.

If you become stressed, you often have a rich imagination of how badly things can turn out, even though nothing serious has actually happened. Stress causes you to continually ruminate about your situation and you become mentally obsessed with your status. You go to bed thinking about your problems and wake up where you left off—thinking about your problems.

Unresolved stress adversely affects your immune system resulting in decreased tolerance to minor infections such as colds or flus. The healing process can be impaired.

Checklist for Stress

Stress is inherent in aviation, but as they say, too much of anything is not good for you. Be aware of and alert for indications of stress in your life, including:

- ✓ Anxiety
- ✓ Irritability
- ✓ Insomnia
- ✓ Depression
- ✓ Trembling, weakness
- ✓ Fixated attention
- ✓ Speech difficulties
- ✓ Forgetfulness
- ✓ Nightmares
- ✓ Impulsive behavior
- ✓ Increased smoking or overeating
- ✓ Inability to concentrate
- ✓ Indigestion
- ✓ Loss of appetite
- ✓ Sweating
- ✓ Emotional tension
- ✓ Headaches
- ✓ Confusion
- ✓ Neck pain
- ✓ Chronically tense muscles
- ✓ Increased self-doubt
- ✓ Proneness to accidents

There are two kinds of stress, acute and chronic. You may experience acute stress if you are anxious about a checkride, an interview for a new job, trying to sell your house, a sick child, or the death of a loved one. It's normal to be stressed-out and anxious, even depressed to some degree. Once the stress is resolved the distress goes away, although we sometimes tend to dwell on the stress beyond that resolution.

Chronic stress occurs when the source of the stress continues without resolution in the near future. Chronic stress might be triggered by a marriage going bad, your company that is failing, flying schedules that disrupt your lifestyle, a challenge by the IRS on your income of several years ago, or a terminally ill family member. This stress can virtually take over your mental processing to the point where concentration is impossible. Some say that the act of flying is therapeutic, but this is false. At best, you are easily distracted. Performance is impaired and you won't be aware of its affects. Chronic stress can lead to illness, poor sleep, and many more symptoms, not the least being fatigue.

The only way to deal with stress is to first recognize that stress is present, which is sometimes difficult. Even after sensing there may be too much unresolved stress, you often feel that you can and must deal with it yourself. This situation has been proven many times to be a great deterrent to actually resolving a stressful situation.

Only by talking about your problems with someone who can be unbiased are stresses identified and overcome. Sometimes professional help is necessary to break through the denial that there is stress affecting your performance and that help is needed. Medication may be necessary while you work at coping with your stress. But this should be used only as a crutch to get you through the healing process.

Current FAA rules require pilots to disclose any treatment by a medical professional on the FAA medical application form. Although this includes therapists counseling someone with stress, you do not have to report this providing the counseling is not drug or alcohol related and you are not on medication. If you are on medication, it's better that you not fly anyway because being on the medication suggests that you are dealing with significant stress. The FAA, indeed everyone, would prefer you to seek help, resolve the stress, and press on. The FAA will not question or deny your seeking help, unless the stress has been allowed to get so severe that it compromises safety.

As a reminder to managing stress, here's a checklist to use—the 5 As:

- Acknowledge that you are under stress and having difficulty coping.
- Accept that you can't deal with or manage your stress by yourself.
- Admit your stress to someone who can help, even to a professional.

- Act on the resolution of your stress and on coping techniques.
- Adhere to the principles used to manage your stress.

Crew Resource Management (CRM)

History has shown that human nature is imperfect and unpredictable. Aviation is a good example. People who choose to fly, whether for fun or profit, are aware of the hazards associated with taking a highly technical machine into the air. Yet, as past (and probably future) accident and incident reports attest, we tend to let human shortcomings interfere with the safety of our endeavors. Just as aircraft have operating limitations, so do pilots and other crewmembers. And individual personalities, egos, attitudes, etc., determine the parameters of each crewmember's effective operating range. *Pilot error* are two words that have been creeping into more and more accident and incident reports in recent years. And although all accidents are tragic, it is difficult to accept that there are accidents in which the information needed to prevent the catastrophe was available but unused. To combat this problem, a relatively new concept has emerged that is steadily becoming a cornerstone of every training environment—crew resource management (CRM).

Crew resource management (formerly called cockpit resource management) is a concept common in aviation, especially commercial aviation with more than one pilot and flight attendants on board. This concept of improving the safety of flight through viewing the crew as a management team and resource, just like any business, is only a few years old. Crew is now considered all resources—pilots and flight attendants, and ground personnel (mechanics, dispatchers, ATC, etc.). Therefore, even single-pilot operations need to consider the techniques and skills of CRM.

The intent in this chapter is not to give comprehensive insight into how to accomplish the goal of improving the management of cockpit and crew resources. New information is coming out all the time from the experiences of companies who are generating their own CRM programs, often under different titles. Articles, books, and seminars are more evident as more is learned about the optimum way to develop, teach, and reinforce the principles of good CRM.

Equally important is the impact of your medical airworthiness—your health and well being—on how you practice management techniques. You can be legal and well trained in CRM as well as experienced and proficient. If you are not medically airworthy and do not respect the issues discussed in this manual, however, then you are not safe simply because you will be unable to function in an acceptable manner.

A long-term National Aeronautics and Space Administration (NASA) research program has identified and shown that nearly 80 percent of air carrier (and other flying) accidents and incidents were related to some form of human factors. A common characteristic is that often the problems encountered by aircrew are associated with poor decision making, inadequate leadership, ineffective communication, and poor management of available resources. Note these are also symptoms of fatigue. It also was noted that training programs placed strong emphasis on the technical aspects of flying, often at the expense or even lack of training in the various types of crew management strategies and techniques that are essential to safe flight operations. Furthermore, over 60 percent of accidents could have been prevented had the crew simply followed company policy and standard operation procedures.

What is CRM?

The basic meaning of CRM is effective and efficient use by crew of all resources available in all phases of flight. This definition needs to be further defined, using traditional terminology common in any situation dealing with people, personalities, and tasks.

The cockpit crew was once considered the sole source of skills and expertise concerning flight and management performance. It is now recognized, however, that the cabin crew (flight attendants, crew as passengers, and available trained passengers) is also essential in a total team, as well as Air Traffic Control (ATC) and company personnel on the ground. The term *resource* pertains to any kind of resource that can be used to safely fly an aircraft, especially under less-than-ideal or unexpected circumstances. The crew, meaning all usable people on board, is the first to be considered. Ground crew, such as dispatchers, meteorologists, mechanics, doctors, ATC, company operations, and other associated personnel are also available resources.

The foundation of any successful business is the management of available resources. The best resources, in abundant supply, are worthless if not properly managed. Companies often fail because of poor management of the resources of people, equipment, and facilities made available to their managers. The same is true on an aircraft. CRM is now recognized in aviation as the way to improve this situation.

Another way of defining management involves the clear understanding of who's in charge, who's responsible, and who's available to manage and use the resources to perform essential tasks, plus a mutual respect for each of these entities.

What's Learned in CRM?

This list can be long when considering specific components of these skills. The following are the key elements of any CRM program.

Decision-Making Skills

Decision-making skills are necessary for all crewmembers, in all situations, whether routine or emergency. This means taking into account the information from the various resources and making an intelligent and professional decision at that moment. Such decisions cannot be effective if poor CRM skills are practiced. You must be confident of the choices and be able to competently communicate the decision.

Leadership Skills

Leadership skills are very individualized. We know there are born leaders and followers. But everyone can be taught the basic qualities of a leader as well as a follower or team player. Such insight is not just for leading others but also for understanding

Decisions, Decisions, Decisions

Crew/Cockpit Resource Management training puts a great deal of emphasis on improving the decision-making process. In addition to organizing and using the resources around him or her, a pilot must be able to use personal resources. A model that is widely followed in the aviation industry provides a means of making orderly decisions. It is the **DECIDE** model, and works as follows:

D—Detect: The pilot detects the fact that a change has occurred which requires attention.
E—Estimate: The pilot estimates the significance of the change to the flight.
C—Choose: The pilot chooses a safe outcome for the flight.
I—Identify: The pilot identifies plausible actions to control change.
D—Do: The pilot acts on the best options.
E—Evaluate: The pilot evaluates the effect of the action on the change and on the progress of the flight.

and respecting the challenges to any and all leaders during all phases of flight. Part of being a team is showing a mutual respect for the leader and a clear understanding of who is ultimately responsible. Additionally, the leader must respect the opinions and observations of the rest of the team.

Communication Skills

Communication is probably the most important factor in any relationship, whether in a marriage; with friends; in clubs, organizations, and companies; or in flying airplanes. Without knowing and comprehending what others are telling you, there is chaos. Failing to communicate is the age-old problem for everyone. Many studies have shown that most people are poor communicators and even worse listeners. If a situation is not clearly understood or heard by all parties, resulting in a common interpretation, then this is a setup for an accident.

Judgment Skills

The use of good judgment is difficult to teach, but it can be done. It must be associated with real-world situations and real-world practice. Attitude, personality, intelligence, and knowledge are key elements, much of which is learned only from experience and maturity along with continued reinforcement of the skills that can be taught. Judgment also comes from applying lessons learned in situations that went wrong. That means keeping an open mind and being willing to change old habits and concepts.

Crew Coordination Skills

Crew coordination eventually comes from applying all these skills and working as an effective team to accomplish the same objective—getting the aircraft off the ground, to its destination, and back on the ground with the passengers thinking your job is simple. This becomes extremely crucial in an emergency where everyone must depend on the resources and skills of each other, without the need to question skills that are expected of each crewmember.

There are other skills that accompany those just defined and they are learned in most CRM courses. These include stress management, respecting situation awareness, problem solving, team management, and other interpersonal skills.

CRM Training Program

A good training program in CRM should include at least three distinct phases: an awareness of the many CRM issues, a practice and feedback of lessons learned using CRM techniques, and a continual reinforcement of CRM principles. CRM, therefore, is defined in a variety of ways. The FAA has a good example:

- CRM is a comprehensive system for improving crew performance.
- CRM is designed for the entire crew population.
- CRM can be extended to all forms of aircrew training.
- CRM concentrates on crewmember attitudes and behaviors and their impact on safety.

- CRM provides an opportunity for individuals to examine their own behavior and make individual decisions on how to improve cockpit teamwork.
- CRM uses the crew as the unit of training.
- CRM is a training program that requires the active participation of all cockpit crewmembers.

The challenge, however, is not simply applying good CRM skills in flight. The challenge is upper management that does not accept CRM. If this is the case, CRM probably will not be as effective. Another challenge is the lack of recognizing the available resources. Flight attendants, for example, when a part of the crew, must be included in any CRM programs. And cockpit crew must work with cabin crew for a mutually effective management of all resources, before incidents occur.

CRM is here to stay, even if it evolves into other programs with different names. The traditional CRM techniques and skills will be used and reinforced long into the future. The sooner you, your crewmates, and other aviation resources begin to incorporate this attitude into flying, the quicker our flying environment will become even safer.

In-Flight Medical Emergencies

10

You're cruising along in the company's jet. Your copilot has finished with her duties and the passengers are engrossed in their conversations. Someone knocks on the cockpit door: "Hey Bill, Frank just banged his head on the cabinet over the sink. He may have knocked himself out but he's okay now. The bad news is he's bleeding like a stuck pig. Can you come back and help us? We don't even know where the bandages are." Your copilot offers to help but you are fast approaching a weather system and ATC is beginning to vector aircraft ahead of you. Both of you need to be in the cockpit for the next 30 minutes. You reply: "We've got our hands full up here for awhile. The first aid kit is below the sink. Do what you can and keep me informed, especially if you think Frank is getting worse."

THERE IS ONLY a minimal chance that you will experience a passenger or crewmember having a medical problem in flight. Hopefully, you are following a good health maintenance program and are sure that you are medically airworthy before you begin your flight. This is not true, however, with passengers and crewmembers who are not following good health maintenance. Medical emergencies do occur in flight and, although uncommon, can be more than just distracting. If someone becomes ill or is injured, there is little you can do in the confines of an aircraft with limited medical aids or insight. There are, however, some basic techniques that can help you deal with the problem and still fly the airplane.

The greatest challenge to you is determining the medical problem and its seriousness. Then it becomes necessary to decide what to do and how quickly you must do it. No matter what medical problem is happening to others in your plane, there is one activity that takes precedence over all others—fly the plane. This sounds simplistic but your urge to deal with the sick or injured is, at best, distracting and it is easy to get caught up in the situation and become removed from the responsibility of flying.

Most medical emergencies can wait until you get the plane on the ground. Declaring an emergency to ATC may require some paperwork afterward, but the controllers are trained to get you to the right airport with the right facilities. They will want to know the extent of the problem, which means you will have to tell them based on your observations and insight. They are able to help you from there, by getting in touch with a doctor or medical emergency personnel. It is better to err on the side of assuming the problem is potentially severe and let the doctor decide if you overreacted.

Often the medical emergency affects someone who can't tell you what's going on. If the emergency involves someone unconscious, then basic cardiopulmonary resuscitation (CPR), if indicated, is about all that you can do, if that. Remember, your role as the pilot is to first fly the plane. If possible, ask someone else on board to help the ill person, and then decide the next step—either press on or head for an emergency airport.

Many flight departments have flight attendants that have access to medical resources and are trained to take action and advise you of the situation. Otherwise, you must know what resources you have onboard, especially before you begin the trip. Even a communication link to organizations that provide in-flight medical advice is a resource.

Short of using basic first aid, most medical emergencies ultimately have to be evaluated by medical professionals. Therefore, insight into basic first aid and what you realistically can do in flight are essential. In larger commercial aircraft, more extensive care can be given, depending on the resources available, such as medical personnel, equipment, space, and a medical kit.

First Aid in Flight

Injuries that require and respond to first aid include lacerations, bumps (contusions), sprains, and broken bones (fractures), suspected or real. Most bleeding can be controlled with pressure over the laceration or bleeding site. Don't waste too much time looking for pressure points unless you know exactly where they are located or if there is extensive or uncontrollable bleeding. Pressure must be maintained for a minimum of 5 minutes for minor cuts. More time is necessary for extensive lacerations that bleed more profusely, as in the scalp.

A bloody nose can be controlled by simply holding the fleshy part of your nose as if you were going to jump into a swimming pool. This pressure also must be maintained for at least 5 minutes, which is a long time, so the time should be confirmed with a timepiece. Techniques such as a cold compress behind the neck or holding a tissue under the nose have little effect, if any. The bleeding usually is from small vessels in the front of the nose and the objective is to put pressure on these vessels.

Sprains, contusions (hard bumps), and suspected fractures are treated the same way, initially. Immobilize the injured part, put ice (if available) over the injury, and wrap it with some protective material. Stabilizing the injured body part is all that is necessary until medical assistance is available.

Burns should be protected until seen by the doctor. Ice or cold water may help. Do not put on any ointments or creams.

First aid kits are usually easy to find in drugstores and contain all that is needed in the short term. It's easy to make your own kit, with Band-Aids, tape, gauze, scissors, elastic bandages, safety pins, Q-tips, tweezers, and a basic first aid manual, all of which can be purchased in any drugstore. Put everything into a plastic bag or small container that is easily accessible. More sophisticated and complete medical kits are available from various organizations. The size of the kit is dependent on the type and length of flying you do.

Remember, all you need to do during a medical emergency before you land is to keep the injured or ill person stable. Try to keep the patient relatively comfortable without disrupting your flying duties. Getting down to an airport is usually only a matter of minutes and will not seriously compromise your ill passenger.

Fainting is a common occurrence in-flight and is often self-limiting. That is, once the person is prone or lying down and blood can get to the brain, recovery often quickly takes place. Try to determine why the person fainted. Was he or she scared,

Contents of Your Personal First Aid Kit
(For use by passengers, not PICs)

- Aspirin, acetaminophen, ibuprofen
- Cold and cough remedies
- Mild laxative
- Antacid
- Sunscreen
- Ice bag (chemically activated)
- Antifungal and itch agents
- Antibacterial cream
- ACE bandages
- Band Aids, cotton swabs, tape
- Large compress
- Tweezers
- Scissors
- Pepto-Bismol
- *Basic First Aid Manual* (Red Cross) or *Boy Scout Manual*

hypoglycemic, hyperventilating, or something more serious (e.g., heart attack, stroke, diabetic collapse). Your insight from the contents of this manual will assist you in determining the extent of the problem, certainly enough to convey to someone else through ATC. If the person does not recover in a few minutes and is not able to tell you what is happening, then obviously you must consider it to be a more serious problem and you are now obligated to seek advice. The size of your aircraft and available space in the cabin determines what you can realistically accomplish.

If the passenger is able to talk, he or she may be able to help you treat the condition. Sometimes, with diabetics, providing some candy or juice helps. If there is no improvement no matter what you do, tell ATC that you have an unconscious or seriously ill passenger that needs immediate medical attention. They will direct you while you fly the plane.

There are some true medical emergencies that do require immediate attention, such as a stroke, heart attack, or diabetic collapse. There is, however, little you can do, especially if the person is unconscious and you are in a small airplane. If O_2 is on board, try to get the mask over the person's mouth and nose. If there still is a problem then CPR should be considered but only after you get clearance for an emergency landing at an airport with medical support. Again, fly the airplane and let someone else work on the passenger. If there is no one else, just fly and try to not be overly disrupted by the onboard medical emergency.

It is very difficult to do CPR, even if you know how, and even in a large aircraft. Hopefully, you will have someone on board to assist if you must perform CPR. You may have to do it yourself or have to guide another passenger by explaining the process.

Choking often occurs during eating or when you are eating in a hurry. A passenger, for example, may try to swallow a large, firm piece of food, such as meat, and it gets stuck in the pharynx. It's fairly obvious what is happening because it often happens during a meal and the passenger is having trouble breathing. He or she is usually holding the neck or pointing to the throat. The person is unable to speak and explain what is happening. If you can get the obstruction out by removing it from the open mouth, then try. The best procedure, however, is the Heimlich maneuver, which also can be difficult to perform in a small airplane. Sudden pain such as from the passage of a kidney stone, a severe headache or toothache, or a gallstone can only be dealt with by getting the plane to an airport.

There are many other scenarios that must be considered, but they are beyond the scope of this manual. Other resources are available. It goes without saying, get medical and keep medical resources on board before you takeoff.

Transporting Ill Passengers

The military has transported sick and injured people for years. They have specially equipped aircraft with adequate medical supplies and equipment. Medical personnel are often on board, including doctors. Civilian air ambulances are very common and are also often well equipped and staffed. These services are professional and competent because they are trained, experienced, and have access to adequate resources.

The flight environment and the restrictions within an airplane can make an existing medical condition worse and even trigger other problems. Therefore, it is often unwise for you to transport known sick people in your aircraft if it is not medically equipped or staffed. Unless the passenger is accompanied by medical personnel with adequate resources and expertise, and there is a release from the company doctor, it would be prudent to defer the trip until you are fully informed of your responsibilities and liabilities if something goes wrong with the passenger, or a known condition worsens.

The reason for this concern is that there are several situations unique to flight that, in most "non-medvac" aircraft, are not suitable for transport of the ill or injured. This includes lack of adequate space to work on a patient, vibration, hypoxia, hyperventilation from scared patients, inability to perform basic tasks such as blood pressure reading, listening to the heart and lungs in noisy conditions, inadequate intravenous fluid and medicine control, and lack of other medical resources. This becomes a real issue if the patient becomes unexpectedly critical during the trip and there are no means to assist. Now you have an emergency that requires you take control as described previously.

The liability of transporting passengers who are already ill or injured in a poorly equipped or staffed airplane also becomes a major factor, as described earlier. The best solution would be to check with a doctor and attorney familiar with aviation law and medical liability before allowing any sick passenger on board.

Basic Survival Techniques

The military requires survival training for all their flightcrews. This topic, however, is rarely discussed in the civilian aviation community because the chances of not being found within a few hours after a crash landing are small. Yet those who fly in and over remote locations, such as the mountains and wilderness areas, are wise to consider the real possibility of having to survive for several days before search and rescue can get there.

When Passengers (Including Pilots) Should Not Fly
(Unless in a medically equipped "air ambulance")

- Recent heart attack
- Uncontrolled hypertension
- Severe heart failure
- Symptomatic cardiac valvular disease
- Uncontrolled cardiac arrhythmia
- Angina
- Severe lung disease
- Recent stroke
- Uncontrolled epilepsy
- Recent skull fracture
- Recent eye surgery
- Sinus or ear congestion
- Late-stage pregnancy
- Uncontrolled diabetes
- Diverticulitis or ulcer
- Brain tumor
- Acute gastroenteritis

Filing flight plans is an obvious initial means of preventing an unacceptable response to a downed aircraft, but there are many who fail to take this simple step and who also are unprepared to survive away from civilization. Emergency locator beacons or other electronic devices are essential.

There are many good manuals and pamphlets regarding how to live off the land and cope with weather extremes. A *Boy Scout Manual* also serves the same purpose and has a wealth of information. All such manuals are available in most bookstores and are strongly recommended to be in your flight bag as a resource for coping with a wide variety of emergencies, including first aid.

There are several priorities that must be dealt with in any survival situation. The first is to tend to injuries, if any, and to ensure that all persons on board are accounted for. The next step is probably the hardest—stop and think. Panic and an unnecessary sense of urgency often cloud your objectives and actions. A plan becomes your strongest asset.

The following high-priority steps can be assigned to each person. Find shelter, especially if the weather is bad or threatening. Get all your supplies in this shelter. Then, look for water. Food is not important at this stage because you can go for days without food. All this should not take long. Then and only then, should you begin to plan for the essentials for continued survival and comfort. Use your first aid manual and whatever supplies you may have, hopefully a survival kit.

Here are a few suggestions for the basic essentials to include in your survival kit: matches that have been sealed with candle wax; a small candle; safety pins; a knife; some thin, pliable wire (for snares); aluminum foil; a small, thin plastic tarp; some fish hooks; nylon line; a plastic whistle; a small compass; a strong balloon (for water container); salt; bouillon cubes; a small flashlight (with batteries covered to prevent contact); a signal mirror; and water purification tablets. All this, plus your first aid kit, can provide the necessary tools to cope with just about any environmental situation.

Keep in mind the word STOP. It stands for Stop, Think, Observe, and Plan. With some minimal preparation, with basic tools, and the self-confidence that survival in extreme environments is possible, your chances of survival are greatly improved.

Aircrew Health Maintenance 11

"If it ain't broke, don't fix it." Or, "I feel fine, why worry." That's what Captain Dave's philosophy was until at age 51, he had his first heart attack. Even though he was back flying one year later, he looks back and realizes that he should have known better. His own father died at 55 of heart disease and his brother had bypass surgery when he was 48. But Dave liked the good life, frequently enjoyed a steak and potatoes with all the fixings, a few cocktails before dinner, and a cigarette with his coffee. In fact, he was so busy enjoying life that he couldn't find time to exercise. And like he said, "I felt fine. I figured that if something happened or I got sick, then I'd deal with it—after it broke. The problem was I didn't know I was broke already! I sure didn't need some doc poking around looking for something wrong or his nurse preaching about getting in shape." A year off the line, scared silly that he wouldn't ever get back flying, got his attention.

PROTECTING YOUR FAA medical certificate is not the only reason that you must be aware of your health. Health is not just a matter of you being productive in your job; safety is an important objective in any flying activity and your health and that of your crew and support personnel must be considered in any safety program. An unhealthy pilot or flight attendant is a potential safety risk. There are plenty of health educational resources, ranging from daily exposure of health issues in newspapers and magazines to a wide variety of good (and not so good) books and manuals available in drugstores, supermarkets, and bookstores.

Health is a topic, more often than not, that is taken for granted. If you do not respect the impact of poor health on your flying status or make a conscious effort to maintain good health, you will be at greater risk of developing a medical problem in the future. And, of course, your FAA medical certificate is based on the status of your health—and you have to periodically prove that to the FAA. Even more significant is that your poor health could make you less than safe during flight, leading to events that show up in incident and accident statistics.

No one can force you be to healthy, except maybe the FAA when they identify an unhealthy and unsafe medical condition and hold up your certification until the problem is resolved. Then you are already behind the power curve of getting back your health and maintaining it. Wouldn't it be a better long-term goal to keep ahead of your health rather than waiting for someone else to challenge your medical certificate or for you to experience a "Boy, that was close!" in flight? Managing your health is no different than managing an investment portfolio—the long-term benefits can only be realized by deliberate and careful investment in your health right now. Here are some suggestions to assist you in your health maintenance.

Nutrition and Diet

Before considering what you should do to maintain your health, it's important to review some basics of nutrition. Granted, there is a lot of information in the press about what you should and shouldn't eat. There is little that has changed, however, in nutritional insight over the past several decades. When you consider the variety of diets, food products, and supplements available, just keep in mind the nutrition basics that you learned in grade school. About the only significant change is in prioritizing the food groups and recognizing the importance of supplements, especially in these days of processed foods.

Basic Food Components

All foods are made up of three basic substances: proteins, carbohydrates, and fats. Other components are vitamins and minerals, but they usually are present in adequate amounts in most balanced, unprocessed diets. Recent studies show there may be more benefit in supplemental vitamins, minerals, and fiber than previously thought.

Protein is the basic substance of all cells in your body and is required by all living things. Approximately 20 percent of your diet should consist of protein. It is a major player in your metabolic processes and tissue growth. During digestion and metabolism, ingested protein is changed into peptides and amino acids, which are the basic building blocks of all proteins. Proteins are commonly found in animal products—meat, fish, poultry, and dairy products. Fruits, vegetables, and grains are another source of protein but to a lesser degree. Ingested proteins cannot be stored and must be replaced every day.

It is a misunderstanding that ingested protein directly replaces lost protein in your body, such as from muscles. All foods are broken down during digestion to simpler components. Then the body forms its own protein in appropriate locations in your body. For example, it is not true that eating more protein builds muscle mass. Proteins in your diet provide the elements for your body to enhance muscle mass. Calories from proteins are also necessary and protein already in your body mass is sometimes used as a source of calories. The body's proteins, however, can be spared by ingesting more fats and carbohydrates. Thus, if sufficient nonprotein calories are not available, then your body's proteins become part of the metabolic process to generate energy.

Fats are a very concentrated (and the primary) source of energy. Only ethanol (the alcohol in beverages) approaches fats as an energy source, but it has no nutritional value. Because your body needs this energy at various times during the day, unused sources are stored in fat cells and tissues. Approximately 25 percent of your diet should be fat. Each person has his or her own rate of use of this energy and ability to store energy in fat. Just controlling calorie intake is not going to be successful in all people. Therein lies the challenge and dilemma of weight control. As with the other food components, ingested fat does not go directly into body fat. It reaches the fat stores via the metabolic route and any leftover calories are stored for future use.

Dietary fats are often classified into three categories: saturated, monounsaturated, and polyunsaturated. Most saturated fats are solid at room temperature, and they are found in animal products, especially beef and pork. A common misconception is that fat is the same as cholesterol.

The majority of a diet should be carbohydrates, approximately 55 percent. Carbohydrates are broken down and metabolized to glucose in your body (also called blood sugar). The function of glucose is to provide immediate sources of energy and it is, therefore, an important body fuel used by muscles and especially the brain.

In addition to calories being stored in your body's fat tissue, some is stored in the liver as glycogen and as a backup if adequate blood sugar is not available. Carbohydrates are no more fattening than fat or proteins—it's still a matter of total calories consumed that determines a healthy diet. This misconception is common even though fat is recognized as having more calories per weight than carbohydrates. Your body metabolizes each component in a different way and at a variable rate, but you cannot maintain an ideal weight solely by avoiding carbohydrates. In fact, that would be unhealthy.

Carbohydrates are found in grains, potatoes, beans, and peas. Other vegetables and fruits have smaller amounts of carbohydrates in the form of starches and sugars. Plain sugar, by the way, is an empty calorie because it does not have other nutrients, vitamins, or minerals associated with these calories.

Another carbohydrate of major importance is fiber. Fiber is essentially carbohydrates that your body cannot digest or break down into usable materials, but they are absorbable. Fiber is important in a balanced diet because it assists in helping move ingested foods and by-products through your GI tract. Lack of fiber leads to constipation. More importantly, absorbable fibers are now proven to be related to reducing cardiac risk factors; lowering cholesterol; raising HDL; lowering blood pressure; and reducing the risks of some colon, prostate, and breast cancers. Weight loss also has been related to increased fiber intake. You need at least 30 grams of absorbable fiber per day.

Vitamins and Minerals

Vitamins and minerals are natural chemicals that are adequately supplied to your body with a basic, balanced diet. Vitamins provide no nutritional or caloric value. They act like a catalyst, assisting in metabolism. Some vitamins are excreted in the urine and therefore need to be replaced, which is usually accomplished by following a nutritious diet. Taking supplemental vitamins does you no harm and may help maintain your health in working conditions that do not always provide the best options for a healthy diet. All vitamins, however, are the same, no matter who manufactures, markets, or sells them.

Calories

Calories are a part of every food that you eat, although some foods contain more calories than others. Calories that are not used by your body are often stored in fat tissues, and some calories are excreted. What happens to calories varies from individual to individual because some people have a metabolic rate that easily gets rid of excess calories. Others have a difficult time losing weight because of their efficient metabolism in using available calories. The rest is stored. Nevertheless, your caloric input is still what decides your ultimate weight. Most overweight people, along with having a low metabolic rate, are simply taking in more calories than needed to function, especially without an exercise program or active lifestyle.

Over time, most trendy diets fail because there is the lack of a maintenance program that keeps caloric intake under control after the initial weight loss. Counting calories, like basic fuel management principles with your airplane, is the best way to keep your weight under control. Furthermore, many diets are not nutritious over the long run. They often are quick fixes at the expense of your body's metabolism, and they generally fail after a few months.

Your body, with usual levels of activity, needs less than 2,000 calories to function, often less than 1,500 per day. Therefore, by counting your calories, keeping track of your intake in a diary, and staying around 1,000 to 1,200 calories per day, you usually experience a weight loss, providing you are active enough to use these calories. As you approach your optimum weight, more calories can be added. This is very simple and it works, but most people need motivation to stick to calorie counting. That's one reason there are so many different and creative methods to losing weight.

Calories Burned per Minute
(For a 170-pound person)

Golf	4.4
Walking (3 mph)	5.3
Swimming	5.3
Calisthenics	7.3
Biking (10 mph)	7.3
Tennis (doubles)	7.5
Aerobic dancing	7.8
Stair climbing	7.9
Handball	10.5
Jogging (5.5 mph)	11.5
Skiing (cross-country)	12.3

Keeping in Shape

Exercise is as important as your diet in your health maintenance program. Exercise means different things to different people. The main objectives are to increase the efficiency of your heart and lungs (aerobic exercise); keep your body's muscles, tendons, and bones toned; assist in a weight control program; and maintain an increased sense of well-being.

The basis of any aerobic exercise is to gradually bring your pulse rate up to a target rate. This target rate is often defined as 220 minus your age and this rate must be maintained for no less than 20 minutes. (Actually, getting up to 85 percent of the level is still beneficial.) Then, you slowly return to your resting pulse. Aerobic exercise is accomplished by jogging, fast walking, biking, cross-country skiing, and swimming. Although jogging may be the most productive form of aerobic exercise in a short period of time, it is not enjoyed by everyone. It is also very hard on your hips and knees. It is important to start some form of exercise program and stick with it for awhile until you find something more to your liking or schedule. A brisk walk is a very good form of exercise. It's better to have some kind of exercise, even if it's for a short period of time. Weekend workouts, however, that push you to your limits are risky.

Try for three times a week or no more than three days between exercise. For aerobic conditioning, working out to achieve more than your maximum heart rate is not safe nor will it gain any more than reaching the 85 percent level. Furthermore, the more you exercise and the more competitive you get, the greater the chance of injury. Injury could keep you from flying while you are healing.

Flight Physicals

Aircraft performance and standards can be measured in absolutes and if you fly the aircraft "by the numbers," it should perform as stated in the manuals. In contrast, the measurements of your body's physiological status are expressed in ranges, not absolutes. For either mechanical or human machines, there are only two ways to determine if something is going wrong or about to fail or fall apart. One way is for you to wait for something to happen (or change) and only then take corrective action (i.e., crisis management). The other way is for you to test the machine periodically to deliberately try to identify a problem, hopefully in the early stages of failing. By identifying the problem you can allow for treatment. For mechanical machines, this strategy of early testing is called a *preventive maintenance program*. For the human body, it's the medical evaluation or physical examination in a health maintenance program.

The FAA requires all pilots to have a periodic medical exam called the flight physical. Without this requirement, it is doubtful that many pilots would seek out their own exams. The reason, of course, is the potential threat that something will be found that could ground you. And this happens. Many pilots reason that as long as they feel good, there really is no need to have further tests to see if anything is wrong. You've heard the saying "If it ain't broke, don't fix it." But how do you determine if you aren't "broke?" This is not the way they would view keeping ahead of their airplane's airworthy status. The difference is the perceived lack of control that you have over the results of your medical evaluation as opposed to the maintenance check of your aircraft.

It is important to recognize what happens in a typical exam because then the threat of losing control should be minimized. It still is a trade-off—looking for something wrong and then unexpectedly finding something wrong. The other challenge is finding something wrong in time to be corrected before the problem becomes unacceptable. The other option, of course, is waiting for something to go wrong. That assumes you really can recognize and admit that something is going wrong! Hopefully you will be able to correct the problem. Therefore, the key to health maintenance is a combination of what was explained earlier—common sense and a prudent lifestyle—and the preventative medical evaluation.

Medical exams, range from a simple overview such as an FAA or insurance physical to a comprehensive medical evaluation that includes several tests and evaluations. Although a basic exam is important, only a comprehensive physical really tells you and your doctor about the overall status of your health. To assist you in determining what you should expect, here is a description of the typical medical exam available to you as a pilot. All medical evaluations consist of a medical history, a physical exam, and a series of tests, followed by a review of the results.

The Medical History

The medical history is the most important part of any medical evaluation, especially for your doctor. How you feel, what has changed in your life, your habits, and your family's medical status all are important clues to your health. But to you as a pilot, this is also the one area where there is a reluctance to be completely candid and thorough. It's that threat thing again, and your denial that a simple symptom could be meaningful or helpful to the doctor. Many of these simple symptoms are valuable in a doctor's overall opinion of your health. It's your understandable rationale, however, to not mention anything unless you think it's significant.

The items of a good, standard medical history review should always be the same. You need to be familiar with the usually asked questions to have consistent answers and explanations. It's especially important if there is a problem in the future. Although some medical evaluations have only a brief review of your medical history, you need to know everything that has happened to you medically. You should keep this information in your personal files. There will be a time in your flying days when you will need to share past information with someone. It makes it easier for everyone to compare data over a period of time to detect changes or trends in health. Another important reason is to show that a condition has always been present and hasn't changed.

Frequently, a medical history question states, "Have you *ever* had a history of ..." That means have you ever had "X" disease, injury, or surgery at *any* time in your life. Even if it was decades ago that you had the problem (e.g., a broken bone, surgery, or hospitalization, etc.), it's important to you and your doctor in the current exam.

It would be wise to have a copy of a typical history form that you have filled out completely, checking with family members to confirm dates, ages, and events of their history as well as yours when you were younger. Check with your personal physician to make sure that everything is adequately evaluated and explained. Keep all this information in your personal files for future use.

Another part of the medical history is called "Review of Systems." This is an explanation of how you currently feel, what symptoms you have, and how you perceive your body is functioning or not functioning. The doctor is interested in any significant pain, discomforts, congestions, aches, dizziness, or other symptom that is not normal for you. Equally important is a change in these feelings—is it better or worse, more often or less often, what makes it worse or better, etc. It's important to realize that what you may think is insignificant may in fact be important to the doctor as he or she considers all the data from the rest of the evaluation. Let the doctor decide what to do with the results. Expect him or her to elaborate on your responses if necessary.

You should have your vaccination records in your file and bring the dates to your doctor. You also will be asked about your habits, such as smoking, drinking alcohol or coffee, exercise, diet, etc. The doctor is not interested just in what you have been doing the last week; he or she also wants to know what you have done in the past, even years ago. Of primary interest is what your lifestyle is like.

The Physical Examination

Like the medical history, the physical is as extensive as the doctor feels it ought to be, often depending on why you are having a physical. For example, a doctor could spend 15 minutes listening to your heart. Often, however, only a few minutes are necessary if there are no abnormal findings. Basically, the doctor is looking, feeling, listening, and smelling for anything that isn't normal or expected.

Usually the doctor starts from the head and works down. Head, neck, chest, abdomen, genitourinary, and extremities will all be examined, including most or all of your orifices. Somewhere in the routine or during the evaluation, the doctor or someone else will check your blood pressure and pulse.

A discussion about high blood pressure is in order because this part of the exam causes the most concern to pilots. Blood pressure is the hydraulic pressure within the arterial system. Normal blood pressure is about 120/80 (remember, there are no absolutes in medicine). The top number (systolic) of this reading is the highest pressure exerted by the heart during a contraction. The lower number (diastolic) is the resting pressure, or the lowest pressure reached in the artery before the next contraction and during the relaxed phase of a heart's muscular activity. Blood pressure does not go to zero between contractions for obvious reasons.

Blood pressure is supposed to be high under conditions of extra work, illness, stress, and, of course, poor health. Blood pressure that remains elevated despite control of these factors is called *hypertension*. Hypertension usually needs treatment or certainly a change in your habits. Usually, a doctor considers starting you on medication if your blood pressure consistently stays above 140/90.

Obviously, for you, every measure must be taken to keep blood pressure under 140/90 by controlling known causes of the elevation. This includes weight reduction if you are overweight, reduction in salt and sodium intake, an exercise program, and control of stress. Some people's blood pressure goes up as soon as they have someone check their blood pressure (i.e., white coat hypertension). If you are one of these hyper-reactors, it would be wise to purchase your own blood-pressure-measuring equipment and keep a written record of your readings. Bring this record with you to your doctor to show that it is normal under usual conditions.

Blood and Urine Tests

Medical technology has become so advanced that a multitude of test results can be achieved from a few tubes of your blood and a small sample of urine. The cost is reasonable enough to warrant full blood profiles (i.e., a series of 25 or more blood test results). Many of the test results, however, are of little value in a screening situation (as opposed to diagnostic). At times, these results of minimal worth are not within acceptable or normal limits nor do they fall within the laboratory's range of acceptable results. The doctor is now faced with the dilemma of what to do next. More tests could be considered even though, realistically, there is little clinical significance to a profile's single, questionable test result. Or the doctor can choose to minimize the medical significance of the result because the rest of the medical evaluation is normal. Regardless, to you as a pilot such test results in the not-normal range could be considered by the flight surgeon and the FAA as being abnormal or unacceptable until proven otherwise. This is another reason to be sure your medical and certification needs are met by competent aeromedical physicians.

Be that as it may, results from blood tests do tell your doctor a great deal about how well your body is functioning. Key blood test results include blood sugar, liver function, kidney function, cholesterol, HDL, LDL, triglycerides, and several other tests relative to your metabolic and heart functions.

When you look at the computer printout of your blood test results, you will notice, again, that absolute, single-number normals are nonexistent. Normal ranges are always stated. These ranges may change as the medical profession gains more knowledge as to the significance of the results relative to your health. For example, the upper limit for acceptable total cholesterol in 1987 was 275. Currently, the level has been reduced to 240 or even 200 in some situations. It is essential that you always have a doctor, preferably an aeromedical doctor, help interpret the results from any test or evaluation.

Normal, Abnormal, Not Normal

It's difficult to convey the significance of a medical evaluation result—is it normal or abnormal? These terms are used commonly in any medical discussion, yet they may have a different meaning to a doctor than they do to you.

There should be little doubt about the meaning of normal. *Normal* means not only an acceptable result but also a result that is perfect, or at least near perfect, for that person; that is, it's in the normal range. But what do you commonly call something that isn't normal? Abnormal? But abnormal could be misleading and have different meanings to someone else and to your doctor.

Abnormal has a varying definition. Abnormal, especially to your doctor, is something that is not only less than normal but also is considered unacceptable, a result or finding that requires further evaluation or treatment. Yet, in the real world it is impossible to be normal in every parameter that is used to define your health. Something that is abnormal is not necessarily unacceptable in your eyes or to the FAA, even though it may be questioned within the medical profession.

For example, using total cholesterol, a value of 200 would be considered normal (as is a blood pressure of 120/80 or vision of 20/20). That doesn't mean that any value above those just stated (or outside the normal range) is abnormal or unacceptable, although your doctor may put that value in an abnormal category until proven to be acceptable.

Thus, when talking to your doctor, something abnormal in his or her mind is already unacceptable. To a nonmedical person, such as you and to the FAA, abnormal may be okay once additional tests are done to prove that the result is okay. So maybe another term should be used by pilots when discussing the results of their exams, e.g., not normal.

Not normal should mean that the value may not be perfect, but it is not really abnormal or unacceptable. Knowing that

Cholesterol and Saturated Fat Content of Common Foods

	Portion *Size*	Chol. *mg*	Sat. Fat *g*	Sat. Fat *Calories*
Butter	1 tbsp	31	7	63
Margarine	1 tbsp	0	2	18
Coconut oil	1 tbsp	0	12	108
Milk, whole	1 cup	33	5	45
Milk, 2%	1 cup	18	3	27
Milk, skim	1 cup	9	1	9
Ice cream	1 cup	59	9	81
Yogurt	1 cup	11	2	18
Ribeye steak	3 oz	70	5	45
Ground beef	3 oz	74	7	63
Poultry (no skin)	3 oz	72	1	9
Fish (sole)	3 oz	59	0.3	3
Shrimp	3 oz	134	0.2	2
Frankfurter	1	27	7	63
Egg	1	274	2	18
Peanut butter	1 tbsp	0	2.8	18

the rest of your medical evaluation is within normal limits now places the less-than-normal value in the acceptable range.

Yes, this is making an issue of a minor point. But note how some people react when they say their cholesterol is 212,vision 20/30, or blood pressure 135/85. Some get very upset and concerned. Pilots are used to relating to absolute terms. If a test result is above (or below) a value that is perceived as being normal, they reason that it is unacceptable. Not true. This is all the more reason to have periodic exams to rule out anything that really is acceptable but may not be normal. You will find this attitude in virtually all aspects of medical tests—weight, sugar in the urine, pulse rate, EKG rhythm, and murmurs, to name a few. It is important, therefore, to fully understand the realistic significance of all medical test results and not be hung up on absolute values.

The Electrocardiogram (EKG or ECG)

The electrocardiogram (EKG or ECG) is a test that measures the internal conduction of an electrical current through your heart muscle. The EKG does not put the current into your body, it measures the current that is made by the cells in the body. The readings come from 12 leads (connections) attached to the chest wall and to your arms and legs, usually by using suction cups or other forms of attachment such as stickies (but not needles). The EKG machine then measures the current and reports the results as tracings on a piece of paper. From this tracing, the doctor can recognize rhythm disturbances, pulse rate, poor O_2 supply to heart muscle, conduction defects (e.g., heart blocks), heart size, and other results about the heart muscle and its conduction system.

The EKG is a valuable screening aid but, like many medical tests, is not a completely accurate, definitive, or reliable diagnostic tool. Thus, the same tracings can be interpreted by different doctors as being normal or abnormal. At times, it is a judgment call, subject to interpretation, and necessitates other opinions. If the reading is considered abnormal, more tests can be done (e.g., exercise EKG or Stress Test, Echo Stress, Thallium scans, etc.) to rule out any pathology that could be the source of the abnormal results. This added data now makes the abnormal result acceptable. It's not normal but it's okay.

The Spirometry Test

Spirometry or *pulmonary function test,* is a measurement of your lung's ability to function, how fast you can exhale, and your air capacity. These are tested by blowing into the machine as quickly and forcefully as you can and then for as long as you can. Some people cannot do this test well because they don't understand how to blow into the machine. Here's a tip. Practice blowing out a match that is held in front of your wide-open mouth (do not purse your lips). Continue to try blowing out the match as you increase the distance from your mouth. The intent of the test is to empty the lungs as quickly as possible and then for as long as possible.

Vision and Hearing Tests

Vision and hearing tests are tests common to all pilots and the significance of their results are explained in chapters 6 and 7, respectively. Because these test results are vital to your safe flight and medical certification, it is imperative that you not take shortcuts. A good eye exam by an ophthalmologist should be done early in your flying, followed with periodic exams as you get older. This exam is in addition to the screening tests with your AME. Hearing is equally important but the shortcut of using the whispered voice test or voice test tells you very little about the quantitative changes in your hearing over time. Audiograms (by using an audiometer) are preferred, and you should have at least one every 1 or 2 years.

Drug Testing

Urine and blood can be tested for just about any chemical or substance known. High-tech equipment can detect minute amounts. Therefore, a company, or government agency can check for anything they want to check for and even determine the level or amount that is considered significant. This includes medication, nicotine, CO, chemicals, alcohol, and drugs.

The Department of Transportation (DOT) and the FAA, in 1989 and 1995, respectively, mandated that certain professional pilots and other people with safety-sensitive jobs be tested for drugs (e.g., cocaine, marijuana, amphetamines, PCP, and opiates). Alcohol is now included in this list because alcohol is a far greater problem than hard drugs. Urine is tested for the presence of these drugs as well as for the level or amount.

This is a two-step process. The first test is for screening the urine for the presence of drugs. It is in this test that several materials and even foods can result in a false positive for a specific drug. In addition, however, the amount of that drug also is measured and must be at a certain level before being noted as positive. If that level is reached, then a confirmatory test is done that involves gas chromatography and mass spectrography, which is virtually 100 percent accurate. These tests define a "footprint" for every known chemical in a series of peaks. No other chemical matches exactly the peaks of another chemical, which means that if the test is positive, then the chemical is undeniably present.

Then the level or amount present is once again determined. This level must be reached before a positive result is reported and is often fairly high, which means that once a test result is reported, not only is the drug present in the urine but also is there at a level that confirms use.

Alcohol testing is now a separate program and part of all training of DOT employers and their employees, including pilots, flight attendants, flight instructors, dispatchers, mechanics, ATC, and other people in safety-sensitive positions. This test is not limited to alcoholic beverages and covers any ingested material that contains alcohol, including medications and mouthwashes. No alcohol should be consumed 8 hours prior to duty nor at all during duty. The testing is done by Breathalyzer, an accurate means of determining the level of alcohol in your body. Violation of these rules results in stiff penalties, ranging from being reported to the FAA to permanent disqualification from the job. Check with your company or organization for further details.

Protecting Your FAA Medical Certificate

12

Fran knew she had reason to be scared when her doctor told her she had a murmur during a routine insurance exam. "Now what I am going to tell my AME? He's sure to ground me! Maybe I shouldn't say anything," she thought to herself. Then she recalled a recent story of how another pilot lost his medical because of a murmur and it took the FAA 6 months to recertify him. Yet, how could she be grounded when she felt so good? She asked her CFI and he wasn't sure what to do and her AME wasn't someone she was willing to ask for advice. Now what? In desperation, she called the FAA, not using her real name, and got the advice she was looking for: get a medical evaluation from a heart specialist and then find an AME who has a reputation of working with the FAA. They even gave her some names to call. She felt better already, knowing she could do something about it.

ONLY A FEW decades ago, the standards for flying as a transport pilot were a good past medical history, freedom from material structural defects, normal judgment of distance, freedom from disease of the ductless glands, and sound pulmonary and cardiovascular systems. That was the old Air Commerce Regulations for certification. Times have changed.

The fear of loosing your medical because of the AME and FAA denying you is often more than the fear of busting a checkride. There is nothing more threatening to you than the required FAA flight physical. The main reason for this perception is that denials do happen and you feel out of control whenever you have to see the AME.

This fear, however, is fueled by many well-embellished and often misleading and erroneous war stories, such as other pilots being denied their medical certification for a minor reason or because the FAA has taken months or years to reach a conclusion. It's no wonder that you dread this annual ordeal and seek out the most lenient AME so as not to rock the boat. In addition, as a pilot worried about losing your medical and your career, you are tempted to or will often deny or minimize medical problems on the application form or when questioned by medical personnel. You assume that the FAA probably won't find out about your problem so why say anything? Ever hear of *Murphy's Law*? Many a pilot has had a disruption of certification because the FAA did find out.

Much of the threat comes from a poor understanding of how the certification process works, relying on crew lounge counsel rather than the facts. In your defense, however, there is little accessible, credible information that explains how the process is supposed to work. Complicating this situation is the recognition that there is plenty of misinformation and poor counsel that tends to lead you into traps, delays, and unnecessary red tape. It needn't be that way.

FAA medical certification is a good example of crisis management by any pilot. As long as you can get by your flight physical, there is little incentive to learn how the FAA medical certification process works—until there is a problem picked up during the exam. This attitude is a source of great stress to you and leads to a feeling of helplessness. Therefore, knowing how the FAA certifies you is essential in removing one more source of stress and distraction in the cockpit. What follows is an overview of the certification process, meant only to show that you do have control, and that the chances of being permanently denied are less than 0.1 percent! For further information and details about specific problems, I recommend that you review my manual, *FAA Medical Certification: Guidelines for Pilots*, third edition, published by Iowa State University Press.

Who's Who?

Here are the key players in the FAA medical certification process.

Aviation Medical Examiner (AME)

The AME is a doctor who is designated by the FAA to examine pilots. He or she is not an employee of the FAA. This doctor can have any medical specialty and often fits you into his or her schedule with the rest of the patients. An AME has no authority to certify you unless everything is normal or acceptable in the examiner's eyes and, of course, by the FAA. Anything suspected as being abnormal or unacceptable has to be reviewed by FAA doctors before you can be certified. AMEs now have more authority, providing they strictly follow FAA guidelines. Each AME has an "AME Guideline" that covers practically all situations, many of which can be certified by the AME.

Flight Surgeon

All aeromedical doctors in the military are called flight surgeons—they have earned their professional wings by being trained in an extensive aviation medicine course. Many AMEs have only minimal knowledge and interest in aviation medicine and certification, although they have been trained in a short FAA course. Civilian flight-surgeon equivalents are AMEs who tend to be more knowledgeable and effective and have the reputation of knowing FAA expectations and procedures. An AME/flight surgeon is someone who specializes in working with pilots and the aviation community in addition to his or her usual medical practice. Flight surgeons are not designated as such in directories but their reputation within the pilot group and even the FAA defines them as a flight surgeon/AME and not as an FAA medical examiner. The only way you can determine what role an AME chooses to play is by talking to other pilots and even the FAA. They know from experience the AMEs who are willing to work with a pilot in complicated or suspicious cases.

Oklahoma City (Oke City)

The FAA's office in Oke City is where all applications for certification (Form 8500-8) go for review by FAA-employed aeromedical doctors. They receive in excess of 2,000 forms per day and all the results are fed into a computer. If anything is abnormal, left blank, or incorrectly filled out, the computer rejects the form, which means it must now be reviewed by a medical person (not necessarily a doctor). If there is doubt as to the medical significance of the exam's results, then one of the FAA doctors gets involved. All forms will be sent electronically after October 1999.

The Oke City level has much more authority to certify, deny, and recertify than in years past. It is also this office that directs a pilot (not the AME) to complete further tests, if indicated, to determine certifiability. Thus, a letter challenging your medical comes directly to you, and not through your AME.

Regional Flight Surgeon

The FAA has several regions around the country. Within each region there is a flight surgeon who has more authority than the AME and can often guide you or your AME in problem cases, especially if clarification is needed about the significance of a problem and what additional tests are to be expected. These doctors still are responsible to Oke City but can sometimes provide an okay to fly while other medical tests are being done.

Federal Air Surgeon

The federal air surgeon is the chief flight surgeon responsible for all civilian aviation medicine issues, including medical certification. Although most of the evaluations and decisions come out of Oke City, the federal air surgeon has the final say in very complex files.

The federal air surgeon and his or her staff in the FAA's Office of Aviation Medicine are responsible for ensuring that the public is protected from unsafe pilots. With adequate documentation of your true health, the FAA tries to certify all pilots if they meet specified standards and are not a significant risk in flight. In fact, denials and deferrals create much more work for the FAA, so there is added incentive to avoid frivolous denials. The federal air surgeon's authority is spelled out in the new regulation on medical standards that went into effect in September 1996.

What's What?

Here are some other terms commonly used in the certification process.

FAR Part 67

FAR Part 67 are the medical regulations that specify aeromedical standards for certification. These standards are usually general compared with military medical standards, which are comprehensively spelled out. This FAR has stayed basically the same for many years, but there are now new regulations and standards that became effective in September 1996.

FAR 61.53

FAR 61.53 is a specific regulation within Part 61 that refers to all pilots, commercial and general. It is noted on the back of your medical certificate as a medical requirement by which you are governed. Specifically, it states: "OPERATIONS DURING A MEDICAL DEFICIENCY. No person may act as pilot in command, or in any other capacity as a required pilot flight crewmember while he has a known medical deficiency, or increase of a known medical deficiency that would make him unable to meet the requirements for his current medical certificate."

Thus, you are not legal if you have any problem that would make you unsafe and unable to pass an FAA flight physical just before your next flight. Because you are probably unaware of the significance or definition of a deficiency, you must find out from someone if you are safe and legal to fly. This often places the burden on you to get correct and realistic guidance before you take off. But from whom? It should be the AME/flight surgeon I have just described or the FAA.

Form 8500

All FAA forms dealing with the application and evaluation for medical certification are labeled as 8500s, or FAA Form 8500. The next number refers to the specific form, whether it's the medical certificate (8500-9), the waiver (8500-15), eye evaluation form (8500-7), or the application for medical certification. It's this application form's number—8500-8—that is usually being referred to when someone states simply "8500." FAA Form 8500-8 is a legal document and you are responsible for its accuracy. If you fail to answer correctly, you will have falsified a legal document and be treated accordingly.

Limitations

There are limitations and requirements stated on the medical certificate that you must follow to be legal. For example, the most common limitation is the need to wear or possess glasses for correction of vision. Thus, the certificate is limited by the requirement to wear or possess glasses. If you are not wearing glasses during flight and you have the limitation that you must wear glasses, then you are in violation of the regulations.

Waiver

The term *waiver* has a double meaning. One is a "Statement of Demonstrated Ability" or SODA; that means that you have demonstrated your ability to fly safely despite the fact that you

You Can Not Fly If You Have

- Had a heart attack
- Passed a kidney stone
- Been unconscious
- Asthma
- An ulcer
- Been diagnosed as chemically dependent
- Been put on long-term prescribed medications
- Diabetes
- Migraine headaches
- A mental disorder requiring medication
- Recently had major surgery or injury
- An abnormal EKG
- Had a stroke
- A heart murmur

UNTIL
THE FAA HAS REVIEWED YOUR MEDICAL FILE
AND
AUTHORIZED YOU TO RETURN TO FLYING.

don't meet absolute standards, such as single eye vision, deficient color vision, missing limbs, and hearing loss, etc. Such a waiver is granted after special practical evaluations or a medical checkride to demonstrate that you are safe. Then it becomes a separate written document that supplements your medical certificate. SODA is now the correct title for these situations.

The other meaning, and one that is used in the new regulations, is the usual terminology expressed when discussing medical problems (i.e., illnesses and diseases and their treatments) and whether or not they are certifiable. If you have a disease initially considered unsafe but can be proven to be safe when flying, then the standards are waived. It's like an exception to the rule because it can be proven that the rule doesn't apply to the pilot who is proven safe. This type of waiver is not a separate written document. Instead, it is a letter stating that after review of the medical file, you meet the intent of federal regulations. This is one reason why medical FARs should not be too specific because it allows the FAA to use their professional discretion as to whether or not you are safe or, at least, an acceptable risk. This letter is not something that you carry with you but you should have a copy in your personal files. The SODA does have to be carried with you and shown to any examiner, if requested.

Typical Certification Scenario

The intent of the FAA medical certification process is to identify any medical, mental, physical, or psychological condition that would make you unsafe. In addition, the FAA is trying to anticipate any abnormal or unsafe conditions that might develop between the time of the current exam and the next required medical evaluation. Problems with this process occur when unexpected abnormals are found during the physical. If the AME doesn't know how to deal with the new finding or doesn't want to become involved, he or she will have the entire application sent to the FAA for review and subsequent instructions.

During this review, which could take a minimum of six weeks just for the FAA to get to your file, you are grounded. It's your lack of control during this delay that is the most threatening to you. You perceive your certificate and your livelihood as being judged by some bureaucratic doctors who are making their decision arbitrarily and you have nothing to say about it. This, in fact, is not the case.

As stated previously, what often happens is that some pilots seek the least-threatening AMEs, but they are also the ones who can be less knowledgeable about the certification process and are unwilling do more than fill in the squares. They certify only those they feel are legal, and send the rest to the FAA to decide. Some AMEs tend to discourage pilots who have a medical problem by saying that the FAA won't certify the problem and often state, "You will never fly again." The fact is that the FAA certifies many conditions often thought by some of the pilot community to be a permanent grounding. Some of these situations include use of hypertension medication, bypass heart surgery, heart attacks, kidney stones, and history of alcoholism. There are airline captains legally flying with a history of these conditions.

In the hands of a competent and knowledgeable AME (the civilian flight surgeon I described previously), any disorder is potentially certifiable if it can be proven to the FAA's satisfaction that the condition will not impair your performance or lead to an unexpected incapacitation in flight, either now or in the near future. Now that's a statement you won't hear very often, but it's true.

Two of the most common, controllable problems leading to delays or even denials are failing to answer all questions (i.e., filling in all the squares) on the front of the application form (FAA Form 8500-8), and not explaining all new affirmative answers or changes from previous exams. The new 8500-8 (revised in 1992) has some different questions and a revised format. Your AME should be able to explain what is required of you. On the back of the form, the AME is supposed to clarify all of your affirmative responses, and fill in his or her portion dealing with the findings during the examination, including test results. The AME then states his or her action—certify, deny, or defer.

Some AMEs will not take the time or effort to further evaluate and explain to the FAA a medical situation that the FAA could question later. The AME has the opportunity in his or her section to satisfy the FAA's expectations. To some AMEs, however, it's simpler, especially when he or she is busy and doesn't want to get involved, to deny you and let the FAA take over the certification or recertification process.

This is why the FAA corresponds with you and not your AME when there is a problem noted or there is an incomplete file. The FAA expects you to initiate and coordinate their requests that are necessary to complete the process. This passing the buck to the FAA becomes a very time-consuming process and certainly is not in your best interest. Many AMEs work with you but there are many others who create more problems for you. In fact, it's my experience that most unnecessary denials are the result of poor AME support, and not the FAA being out to get you. (Fig. 12-1).

Ideal Certification Process

The key to an efficient certification process, whether you are healthy or not, is to work with a knowledgeable AME, such as an AME/civilian flight surgeon. Unnecessary delays and red tape do not have to occur. As noted previously, these AMEs anticipate what the FAA requires for further testing, arrange for the evaluations, work up a completed file, may discuss your case with one of the FAA doctors, and then, and only then, submit the file for FAA approval. A major cause of unnecessary delays is having reports from several different doctors arriving in Oke City at different times. It's best that a complete file be prepared before submission so that everything is together when it reaches an FAA doctor's desk.

In less complex situations, an AME/flight surgeon can often be authorized by the FAA, sometimes by phone, to certify you based on the results of the evaluation. The FAA also respects these AMEs, knows they have a reputation of being thorough and professional, and often relies on their judgment to make a final decision. Even the FAA in Oke City or their regional flight surgeon can help or give you guidance. Call them, anonymously. Despite their reputation among pilots and the common joke about their purpose in life, they are paid to help you, if you are willing to comply with the FAA's expectations (Fig. 12-2).

Fig. 12-1 Improperly managed certification sequence.

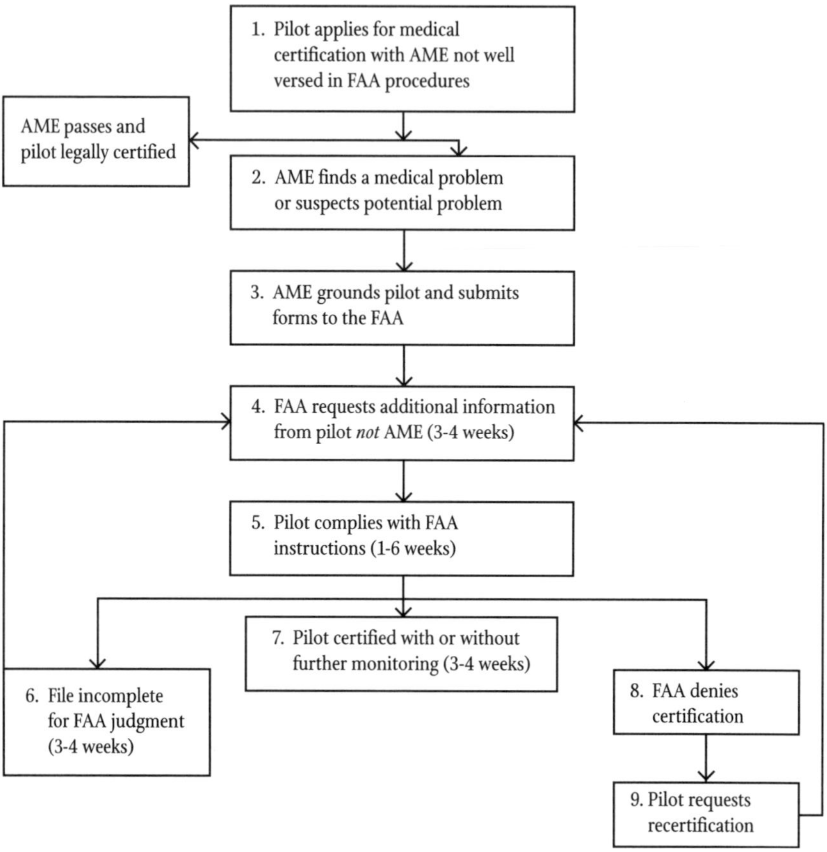

COMMENTS:

#1. The typical AME is not highly knowledgeable regarding expeditious handling of problem certifications.

#2. Often AME does not tell pilot significance of findings—allows FAA to be "bad guy" and inform pilot he is grounded.

#3. Often prematurely submits report to FAA.

#4. FAA requires additional medical information to reconsider a pilot's fitness.

#5. Pilot sometimes left on his own to work with specialists and handle additional paperwork required by FAA.

#6. Because of misunderstanding concerning intent of further evaluation and requirements, FAA requests further data, pilot is back at box 4.

#8,9. By this point pilot often finds himself trying to coordinate and achieve cooperation from 3 entities: the original AME, any specialists who have entered the picture, and the FAA.

Key to improperly handled sequence is not knowing and properly *anticipating* the FAA needs in *advance* of their requests. Tremendous amounts of time can be lost waiting for the FAA to respond to previous paperwork submission—only to learn more paperwork is necessary.

Fig. 12-2 Properly managed certification sequence.

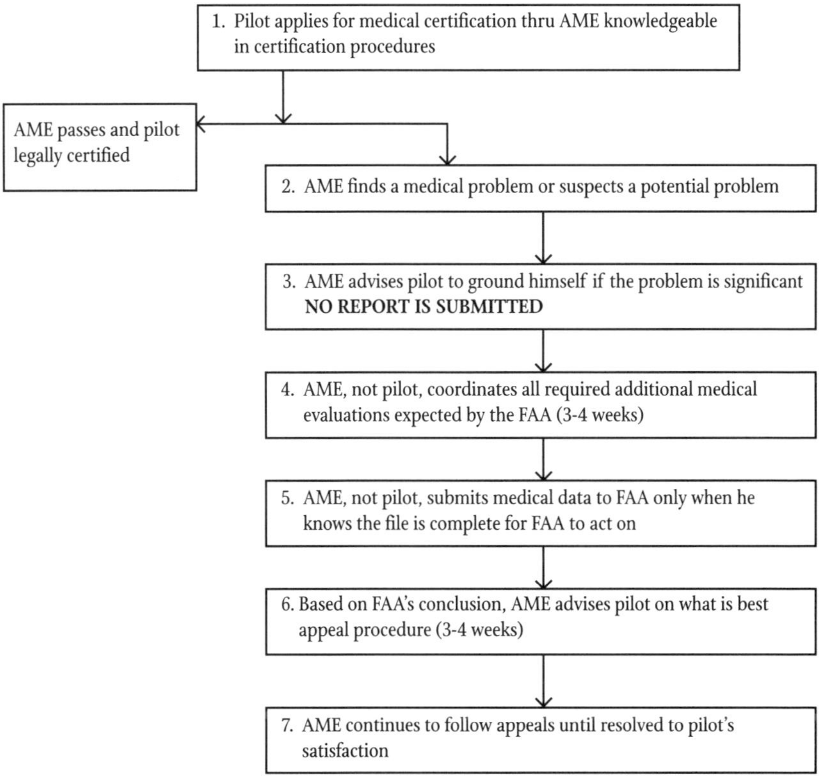

COMMENTS:

#1. This is the key to success of control: that the AME is knowledgeable in the certification process and aviation medicine, and is experienced in working with the FAA in protecting the healthy pilot's medical certificate.

#2. AME will try to anticipate potential problems which can be resolved without compromising your responsibilities as a pilot.

#3. This is the second key to success: No report is made to the FAA until both the AME and pilot are satisfied with the file. If pilot's condition is not significant, pilot continues to fly.

#4. AME can make appointments with other specialists and already knows what the FAA will require for further evaluation. There is no need to wait for FAA's direction.

#5. AME submits entire file to FAA, with cover letter, rather than making the FAA the coordinator of the varied medical reports. AME may also alert FAA about coming file.

#6. AME can then determine what courses of action to follow once everyone knows what is necessary to satisfy FAA requirements.

#7 The AME should commit himself to the pilot to assist him through the entire appeals process and explain why such actions are necessary.

Grounded

The most feared word in aviation is *grounded,* meaning the same as *denial.* It's the word used when the FAA feels you have a medical condition that isn't safe.

There are some conditions that ground you for a few days or weeks(e.g., a bad flu, a broken bone, a sprain, appendicitis) and you go back flying when you and your doctor agree that you have no restrictions to any activities. There are other conditions, more serious, that require approval from the FAA before returning to the flight deck. Such conditions include the passing of a kidney stone, a stomach ulcer, a bleeding ulcer, a concussion, and major surgery. Check the front of the 8500-8 for the disorders on which the FAA will want more information. Still other medical problems (i.e., the 15 mandatory denials) usually begin as a denial but often can be reconsidered.

A denial, contrary to what many think, is never final. The FAA will always consider additional information from additional tests and medical opinions. The passage of time without progression of the medical problem also is taken into consideration. Therefore, if you want to return to flying, you should continue to pursue additional data with the help of an AME/flight surgeon to prove you are safe. If you have a condition that is controllable or curable, then it is up to you to work at your health.

There are several medical conditions that require mandatory denial at the time of discovery of the problem. These include a character or behavior disorder severe enough to be unsafe, a psychosis, severe personality disorder, bipolar disorder, substance dependence, substance abuse, epilepsy, disturbance

Medical Certification Key Points

- A denial is never final unless you accept it as final.
- If you are fit to fly, the FAA should certify you.
- If you don't fly, no report need be sent to the FAA.
- Seek competent advice before requesting recertification.

of consciousness without satisfactory explanation, transient loss of nervous system functions, heart attack, angina, significant coronary heart disease, cardiac valve replacement, permanent cardiac pacemaker implant, heart replacement, and diabetes requiring any medication. It's also important to recognize that this refers to a "history of ... ," which means that, if at any time in your life you have had any of these conditions, denial is mandatory by every AME and the FAA.

That's the bad news. The good news is that the federal air surgeon or his or her designated doctors, through the medical regulation FAR 67.19, can special issue a certificate (now called an authorization), even for the mandatory denials, if it can be proven that the condition, treated or untreated, will not be a safety issue. This regulation is worth reading.

Getting Your Medical Back

If you are denied for any reason, from failing to submit a completed application to having a serious medical condition, the process is the same and has been explained in general terms previously. In the hands of a competent and helpful AME/flight surgeon, additional tests are accomplished, a file compiled, and discussions held with the FAA doctors.

The FAA expects certain minimum tests to be done. Some personal nonaviation doctors may say that such tests are not necessary or assume that if they say you are okay to fly that the FAA should accept their opinion. In most cases, however, the FAA will still require these evaluations and will not consider certification until they are done. The FAA will not accept the doctor's unproven opinion saying that what you have is not significant. Unless there is objective evidence to back up that opinion, the FAA cannot act favorably. It may take several attempts with new information to convince the FAA that you are safe. The passage of time is often necessary just to ensure that you will not have a recurrence or progression of your disorder.

As mentioned, FAR 61.53,which deals with your responsibility to be medically qualified every time you fly, is in effect only when you fly. This is a simplistic observation but it is the key to you keeping control during the recertification process. Providing you are working with a flight surgeon/AME and in the process of evaluating your condition, then nothing has to be reported to the FAA as long as you don't fly. In other words, you ground yourself. This allows you the time to complete your evaluations and precludes premature submission of incomplete files to the FAA. The sense of urgency, which inevitably results in very lengthy and often unsatisfactory delays, is relieved because nothing needs to be submitted until you are ready. You remain in control.

A responsible pilot's fear is not just that something will be found during a medical exam. It's the feeling that the condition must be reported to the FAA immediately, leading to the familiar war stories of prolonged and unfair results. If you don't fly and the AME respects you and your commitment, then you and the AME have breathing room to work out the problem before anything is reported.

In summary, if you are willing to accept the responsibility of being familiar with the FAA certification process and to work with an AME/flight surgeon while you are healthy and before any problem unexpectedly develops (avoiding crisis management), then there is a less threatening situation whenever the time comes for the FAA or company physical. Waiting for something to happen, going to an AME who gives a "pink and breathing" physical, and being informed only through crew lounge counsel will lead to your own bona fide war story of you losing your medical for unexpected reasons. Look for a competent AME/flight surgeon now by checking around. Don't wait until a problem develops. Then practice good health maintenance.

I encourage you to review my manual, *FAA Medical Certification: Guidelines for Pilots*, third edition. It covers all the new regulations, standards, and FAA expectations, and provides a complete guide for certification and recovery of denied medicals plus an abridged version of the *AME's Guide*. It is available from Iowa State University Press.

Appendix

Frequently Asked Questions by Flight Attendants

This manual focuses on topics associated with the physiology of flight for cockpit crew (i.e., pilots and copilots), but there are some unique issues related to the cabin crew (i.e., flight attendants). Here are a few frequently asked questions by flight attendants.

Q. How congested is too congested to fly?
A. Unlike pilots whose impaired performance has a direct impact on safe flight, as flight attendants you have more latitude to accept minor impairment, such as congestion from a cold or hay fever. The preflight use of decongestants and long-acting nose sprays will still allow you to function. It's still a judgment call if you are unable to clear your ears or you feel ill.

Q. Am I held to the same rules as cockpit crew regarding the use of drugs?
A. The answer has two parts. The use of drugs that are part of the drug testing program affects all personnel in safety-sensitive jobs, including flight attendants. There is no list of medications that are disqualifying. Pilots essentially can't use any medications unless accepted and approved by the FAA. Common sense regarding side effects and the reason for needing the medication dictates if your performance as a flight attendant is significantly compromised.

Q. What drugs or measures can I use to deal with fatigue and jet lag?
A. There really aren't any, other than caffeine and sleeping pills and the suggestions described in Chapter 8 on fatigue. Because there are no special rules, however, the use of prescription sleep medication is more acceptable than for pilots.

Q. If I'm pregnant, will flying affect my health or the health of my unborn child?
A. No, because the unborn child is very well protected in the uterus, probably more so than you. Having said that, there remains some controversy within the aeromedical community regarding radiation exposure in the first few months of pregnancy. The most realistic answer, therefore, is to check with your doctor.

Q. Am I more at risk in the cabin than in the cockpit for radiation exposure?
A. No, because the protection from the aircraft hull and plastic windows is the same for all on board. Most studies show that there is probably less exposure than that experienced from background radiation on the ground. There is, however, still some potential concern during early pregnancy and you should check with your personal physician for more information.

Q. Will my menstrual cycles be affected by flying?
A. Not directly from flying; however, the flight schedule, jet lag, trip length, and other disruptions to your body's usual circadian rhythms can disrupt a cycle.

Q. Is the quality of the air in the cabin going to affect me more than if I were in the cockpit?
A. The same air quality exists throughout the aircraft, although the cockpits in some aircraft have their own circulation system. In most modern high-altitude jets, the air is recirculated and filtered many times each hour, keeping the air quality better than in many offices. The same filtering, especially in the newer aircraft, can remove most infectious particles. Because of dehydration from the inherent low humidity, you must drink plenty of water in flight as described in Chapter 4 on dehydration.

Q. Can I catch diseases such as hepatitis when collecting food trays from passengers?
A. Most common serious infections have to be either directly inhaled or ingested, or enter through a break in the skin. Com-

mon-sense hygiene, frequent hand washing, and care in what you eat and drink should reduce any risk of becoming infected.

Q. Are there immunizations that I should have if I travel abroad?
A. That depends on the countries to which you travel because each one has its own endemic diseases. You should check with a clinic that has travel medicine doctors for which immunizations are recommended. Such information is also available from the Centers for Disease Control (CDCs) or the U.S. Department of Health as well as their web sites.

Q. I seem to develop a dry cough on long flights. Why?
A. There are several possible causes for a dry cough, some of which depend on the type of aircraft and the flight altitude. Generally, the higher the aircraft flies, the greater the risk of significant dehydration from dry air, leading to irritated mucous membranes, and exposure to ozone. Many aircraft have ozone filters, but in those that don't, the irritation increases because of your increased activity within the cabin. You also may become more fatigued as a result of being hypoxic. You must pace your activities relative to the degree of fatigue.

Most of the health concerns that you may have about flight are explained in this book. Most cabin crews, however, don't have the protection of rules and policy regarding duty time, medication, meals, etc., and must look to company policy for guidance and protection. Furthermore, the level of activity and the varied tasks that you are expected to accomplish amplify many of the conditions explained in this book for cockpit crew. As a flight attendant, you are encouraged to become knowledgeable about these situations, do your homework, and relate it to preservation of performance and safety. Then, convince your company management to incorporate the same types of protection as there is for pilots, taking into consideration your unique job in flight.

Index

D